African Responses to HIV/AIDS

African Responses to HIV/AIDS

Between Speech and Action

Edited by
Segun Ige and Tim Quinlan

UNIVERSITY OF KwaZulu-Natal Press

Published in 2012 by University of KwaZulu-Natal Press
Private Bag X01
Scottsville, 3209
South Africa
Email: books@ukzn.ac.za
Website: www.uknznpress.co.za

© University of KwaZulu-Natal

ISBN: 978-1-86914-233-9

Managing editor: Sally Hines
Editor: Alison Lockhart
Proofreader: Catherine Rich
Typesetter: Patricia Comrie
Indexer: Abdul S. Bemath
Cover design: MDesign
Cover photograph: Eric Miller / Independent Contributors / Africa Media / Online

Printed and bound by Intrepid Printers - 7067

When one interrogates issues of place, situation, milieu, and occasion that involve African people as participants, it is important to look for the concept of agency as opposed to dis-agency. We say that one has found dis-agency in every situation where the African is dismissed as a player or actor within his or her own world. I am fundamentally committed to the view that African people must be seen as agents in economic, cultural, political, and social terms. What we can argue about in any intellectual discourse is the degree to which Africans are weak or strong agents, but there should not be any question that agency exists. When agency does not exist we have a condition of marginality, and the worst form of marginality is to be marginal in your own story.

Molefe Kete Ashante, *An Afrocentric Manifesto*

Contents

Acknowledgements

This project received support from many individuals, including the entire staff of the Health Economics and HIV/AIDS Research Division (HEARD) at the University of KwaZulu-Natal, Durban. We owe a debt of gratitude to Professor Alan Whiteside and to Obed Qulo who were instrumental in securing funding for this project. HEARD's project administration section (Wilondja Muzumbukilwa, Julius Piko Mkhize and Sylvester Louis) worked tirelessly, especially during the symposium and the review workshops. Members of HEARD's finance team, Nalini Sharma, Vani Venkatas and Nadia Govender, should also be commended for their timely remittances and problem-solving skills. Fehmidah Khan helped with the preparation of contracts and management of logistics.

This project was supported by the Rockefeller Brothers Fund as well as HEARD's core funders, including the Swedish International Development Cooperation Agency (SIDA), the Norwegian Ministry of Foreign Affairs, the United Kingdom's Department for International Development (DFID), the Joint United Nations Programme on HIV/AIDS (UNAIDS), Irish Aid and the Royal Netherlands Embassy.

All the contributors and the internal editorial review committee (including Professor Ademola Ajuwon and Professor Paul Nkwi) should be highly commended for their timely submissions and efficiency. Scott Naysmith and Clara Rubicam should be thanked for their encouragement and sustained interest in this project. Our gratitude also goes to Mike Rogan who served as researcher, and to our families for the support and love shown throughout this project.

Finally, we would also like to thank the staff of UKZN Press, publisher Debra Primo and her editors, for the attention they gave to this volume.

Segun Ige and Tim Quinlan

Abbreviations

ABC	Abstain, Be Faithful, Condomise
ABMPH	African Broadcast Media Partnership Against HIV/AIDS
AIDSCOM	AIDS Public Health Communication Project
ALCS	Association de Lutte contre le SIDA (Association for the Fight against AIDS)
AMJCS	Association Marocaine des Jeunes contre le SIDA (Moroccan Association of the Youth against AIDS)
AMSED	Association Marocaine de Solidarité et de Développement (Moroccan Association of Solidarity and Development)
ANC	African National Congress
ARV	antiretroviral
ASRP	African Social Research Program
ASSA	Actuarial Society of South Africa
AU	African Union
CBO	community-based organisation
CCM	Country Co-ordinating Mechanism
CSO	civil society organisation
DFID	Department for International Development
EAC	East African Community
FGC	female genital cutting
GEAR	Growth, Employment and Redistribution
GFATM	The Global Fund to Fight AIDS, Tuberculosis and Malaria

GRTS	Gambian Radio and Television Services
HEARD	Health Economics and HIV/AIDS Research Division
HSRC	Human Sciences Research Council
INDH	National Initiative for Human Development
LM-MST	Ligue Marocaine de Lutte contre les MST (Moroccan League for the Fight against STIs)
MCPs	multiple concurrent sexual partners
MRC	Medical Research Council
MSF	Médicins sans Frontières (Doctors without Borders)
MSM	men who have sex with men
NAC	National AIDS Council
NACOSA	National AIDS Committee of South Africa
NAS	National AIDS Secretariat
NGO	non-governmental organisation
NSP	National Strategic Plan
OAU	Organisation of African Unity
OPALS	Pan-African Organization against AIDS
PCR	polymerase chain reaction
PEPFAR	President's Emergency Plan for AIDS Relief
PLWHA	people living with HIV/AIDS
PMTCT	prevention of mother-to-child transmission
RDP	Reconstruction and Development Programme
RVTH	Royal Victoria Teaching Hospital
SADC	Southern African Development Community
SANAC	South African National AIDS Council
SIDA	Swedish International Development Cooperation Agency
SIDACTION	Ensemble contre le SIDA/Collective against AIDS
STD	sexually transmitted disease
STI	sexually transmitted infection
SYSS	Santa Yalla Support Society
TAC	Treatment Action Campaign

TCAHZa	Trust for Collective Action Against HIV and AIDS in Zambia
UNAIDS	Joint United Nations Programme on HIV/AIDS
UNFPA	United Nations Population Fund
UNGASS	United Nations General Assembly Special Session
VCT	voluntary counselling and testing
WHO	World Health Organization
ZNBC	Zambia National Broadcasting Corporation

Introduction

HIV/AIDS Rhetoric in Africa

Segun Ige and Tim Quinlan

Nearly thirty years after the discovery of HIV/AIDS, Africa epitomises the tragedies that the virus has wrought upon human welfare. African explanations as to why interventions to curb the pandemic have not worked range from government ineptitude to a lack of resources – the latter frequently favoured by governments. Our contention is that this kind of rhetoric amounts to a travesty because it indicates an unacknowledged but widespread underlying attitude among African governments, who were and still are ambivalent about their citizens' right to life. This is the theme of this book.

This project commenced with a symposium in 2007, a time when the South African Parliament was grappling with a growing tension surrounding ministerial conduct, as well as difficult policy options relating to the mass provision of antiretroviral (ARV) medicines. The latter led to a polarisation between government and civil society, as was also the case in most countries elsewhere on the continent. An observation of the deliberations, debates and presentations in the South African Parliament led to the conceptualisation of a book project that would factor in the role of rhetoric in the politics and the state's management of HIV/AIDS, not only in South Africa, but also the rest of Africa. This project takes into account the many conferences that have been held on HIV/AIDS, the numerous deliberative rhetorical transactions that have taken place in different political arenas, practical humanitarian interventions and multidisciplinary discursive formations around HIV/AIDS. While there are many debates and dialogues on the subject of the pandemic, none of the works that have been produced, particularly those that relate to the African condition, have employed a rhetorical perspective. There is therefore a need to interface discourse with state politics and management of HIV/AIDS, particularly from a pan-African perspective. It is important to say that the foregoing merely served as a platform for conceptualising this book, some countries (such as South Africa) later changed their policies on HIV/AIDS before this project was finalised.

An attempt to understand the patterns of state responses in Africa should not be seen as merely an academic exercise nor is it a deliberate confrontation with the African ruling elite. It is rather a way of paying due attention to the lessons that African states need to learn from the HIV/AIDS experience. One distinctive element of the pandemic has been its ability to provide societies with a common agenda and, so far, Africa has not been an exception. While each country has its own methods for setting the agenda for public policy, there remains a concerted effort among African governments to adequately maintain and sustain intervention programmes by eliminating factors that threaten quality implementation. The complications that arise from poor management of public affairs are therefore arguably as threatening to the stability of African states as HIV/AIDS itself.

For a protracted period of time, African states and their citizens have engaged in rancorous debates over HIV/AIDS issues and in some cases there have been sharp divisions that have led to litigation, especially between government and civil society organisations. The strength of some nation states, governments and even science was tested beyond their capacity and skills to manage a full-blown epidemic. The socio-political contestation over the interaction of the body, the disease and medicines became aggravated and partnerships and fallouts have occurred in numerous spheres and forms.

Our focus here is less on popular criticism of government responses to HIV/AIDS and more on the ambivalence in government responses. We refer here to the equivocation and occasional denial of HIV/AIDS as a human catastrophe in the public statements of Africa's political leaders alongside the proclamation of policies and strategies to confront the pandemic, supported by massive international funding and public interest. We refer also to the multitude of deaths and public condemnation of the failures of governments alongside perceptions and records of successful interventions in some countries to reduce the spread of HIV/AIDS. These are dissonances in the history of the pandemic in Africa that we sought to address when conceiving this book.

We were cautious in our planning as we recognised the difficulties of presenting a singular argument; there would inevitably be counter-evidence to any argument and evidence of an identifiable trend or pattern in political discourses and events. There are also apparent commonalities throughout Africa in public discourses, often apparent in the anger, confusion and frustration voiced in many quarters about the distress caused by the pandemic. Likewise, there has been the development of grand strategies and frameworks for intervention in different sub-populations, reflected in similar national policies and structures, as a result of global initiatives and guided by international agencies such as the World Health Organization (WHO) and the agencies of the United Nations. However, there is as much variation within and between national and local perspectives and responses in Africa as there is discernable commonality.

There was, nonetheless, a beguiling imperative to present an 'African perspective', in the face of the seeming dominance of ideas, explanations and design of interventions emanating from these international agencies, which is often expressed in terms of a division between the global North and South. We refer here to the host of public and private debates in Africa about the power of political and scientific agencies in the North to dictate to Africans how to solve the problem of HIV/AIDS and the consequences in terms of how African views are ignored, even silenced on occasion. We preferred, however, to see these debates as projections of public frustration with the challenges posed by the pandemic. We were also well aware that at best we could present African perspectives in view of the diverse histories of HIV/AIDS in Africa and, if organised thematically, the book could present valuable insights into the patterns within diversity and commonality of what has happened and is happening on the continent.

Consequently, our approach was to ask a range of African scholars to consider the proposition about the ambivalence of African governments with regard to HIV/AIDS on the basis of their work and experience in Africa. The unifying theme was to be the 'rhetoric of HIV/AIDS in Africa'. We felt that this theme would underpin a book which was attempting to cover a very large topic: the politics and management of HIV/AIDS in Africa. It would guide the authors to focus on how and why people have persuaded others, tried to persuade and have been persuaded to act in particular ways in response to the pandemic. This is the sense in which we use the term 'rhetoric'.

For us, rhetoric is the critical ingredient within and between speech and action. Revealing the ways of persuasion used in relation to any particular context or issue is a vital step for understanding why and how things happen. We do not view rhetoric in the popular sense of 'myth' or arguments that are divorced from reality. We do take into account, however, the fact that there is often little correspondence between the rhetoric of politicians and governments and their actions. Rhetoric is inevitably subjective, being subject to particular conditions, contests for power and limitations of knowledge. As readers will see in the following chapters, the rhetoric of HIV/AIDS in Africa and in governments' actions is diverse. It is occasionally logical and effective in terms of leading to systemic interventions that improve the welfare of people. It is often full of contradictions and sometimes absurd; these factors being the grist for many of the chapters' critiques of governments' perspectives and actions because of the tragic consequences for people infected and affected by HIV/AIDS. The purpose here is to draw lessons for future thinking and planning of interventions in Africa by illustrating the positive and negative consequences of the rhetoric of HIV/AIDS on the continent. This quote from St Augustine helps to describe our purpose more eloquently:

He likes what you promise, fears what you say is imminent, hates what you censure, embraces what you commend, regrets whatever you built up as regrettable, rejoices at what you say is cause for rejoicing, sympathises with those whose wretchedness your words bring before his very eyes, shuns those whom you admonish him to shun . . . and in whatever other ways your high eloquence can affect the minds of your hearers, bringing them not merely to know what should be done, but to do what they know should be done (in Burke 1950: 50).

* * *

In Chapter 1, Segun Ige and Tim Quinlan provide a framework for the book's criticism of African governments' responses to the HIV/AIDS pandemic. They examine patterns in national responses since the 1980s to show the poverty of executive leadership and the limitations imposed on citizens' rights to healthcare. The key concepts with regard to the variable efficacy of national responses to the pandemic are transformational and incidental leadership. With regard to citizens' rights, in the context of general ambivalence of African heads of state to the welfare of their citizens, Ige and Quinlan show how and why states see their citizens as 'enemies'.

Chapters 2, 3 and 4 present positive constructions of leadership in Africa. These chapters illustrate the practice of transformational leadership. However, Chapter 4 also introduces the negative values of incidental leadership, illustrated in subsequent chapters by the constraints that governments have imposed upon civil society organisations' innovative responses to HIV/AIDS.

In Chapter 2, Judith Flick discusses an exercise in Zambia that sought to define and cultivate the type of leadership required to contain the pandemic. She describes the theory and practice of this project, which entails personal journeys inward that reflect the need for leaders to look closely at what is happening in their own societies.

In Chapter 3, Fatima Harrak describes the leadership in Morocco that has enabled it to sustain systemic and successful initiatives to contain the spread of HIV/AIDS. Harrak shows that Morocco endorsed internationally sanctioned strategies but, equally, set priorities, monitored progress and used locally relevant means to mobilise people.

In Chapter 4, Shauna Mottiar addresses the vital role that civil society organisations in South Africa have played in developing innovative responses to HIV/AIDS. Her analysis highlights the transformative vision that the country's Constitution provides alongside the constraining role of the government's efforts to contain its HIV/AIDS epidemic.

Chapters 5 and 6 present two notorious examples of poor leadership in Africa and the disastrous effects on their respective countries. The cases are diametrically different. One case describes presidential suspicion of science in favour of an 'African' perspective, of which the effect was curtailing the development of an effective national response. The other case describes presidential manipulation of science and African traditional healing to serve personal claims of an ability to cure HIV/AIDS.

In Chapter 5, John-Eudes Lengwe Kunda and Keyan Tomaselli explore the ideological underpinnings of the 'denialist' agenda that characterised the political stance of Thabo Mbeki, South Africa's president for much of the 2000s (till 2008). They highlight the reactionary nature of the president's ideology, which had two core components: 'resistance to imperialism' and 'African Renaissance'. They show, on the one hand, how this ideology created a divide between science and the state and, on the other, the devastating effects on people's lives.

In Chapter 6, Stella Nyanzi examines how The Gambia's president, Yahya Jammeh manipulated state authority to conjoin science and the state in service of his personal claims of an ability as an Islamic healer to cure HIV/AIDS. Her detailed analysis uncovers the many layers of conflicts and compromise that have threatened the development of an effective national response to HIV/AIDS.

Chapters 7 and 8 engage with interpretations of the sexual transmission of HIV/AIDS in Africa. They examine this issue in very different ways but, at root, they highlight the importance of national responses being based on evidence related to context.

In Chapter 7, Paul Nchoji Nkwi and H. Russell Bernard dispel popular and tacitly racist judgements that the high prevalence of HIV/ AIDS in Africa is due to specifically African sexual practices. They use a continental survey to show clearly what science has to say about the heterosexual transmission of the virus in Africa, about the insignificant role of specifically African sexual practices and the effectiveness of an indigenous intervention, which originated in Uganda and is commonly known as ABC (Abstain, Be Faithful, Condomise).

In Chapter 8, Getnet Tadele confronts the myth that homosexuality is not 'an African phenomenon'. He presents a detailed analysis of the experiences of Ethiopian men who have sex with men (MSM). His analysis shows how social stigma is internalised by these men, with one effect being the perpetuation of the erroneous belief amongst them that 'gays' are insulated from HIV. His analysis also shows how state prosecution of homosexuality closes a space for constructive HIV/AIDS interventions.

Chapters 9 and 10 provide assessments that serve as a backdrop to the detailed case studies of the preceding chapters. In Chapter 9, Ademola Ajuwon provides an overview of how race and ethnicity are ingrained in public and scientific discourse on HIV/AIDS. He examines the confusion that these concepts create, including the potential and actual abuse of them in scientific discourse about the diseases. In Chapter 10, Warren Parker presents the political economy of HIV/ AIDS in South Africa. He discusses the epidemiology of the disease in relation to inequalities of power. He shows how and why social mobilisation within communities is both necessary and possible, while also highlighting the dangers of national responses that adhere to internationally sound strategies but do not incorporate clear priorities and considerations of the local context.

What the chapters in this book have accomplished is the reinvigoration of the notion that nation states survive as discursive entities and the rhetorical processes upon which state policies are based require attention. The HIV/AIDS crisis experienced by most African countries was due to not simply medical or any other singular factor, but the very means by which nations are established, consolidated and maintained: speech followed by appropriate action.

Reference

Burke, K. 1950. *A Rhetoric of Motives*. Berkeley: University of California Press.

1

HIV/AIDS and the State

A Critique of Leadership in Africa

Segun Ige and Tim Quinlan

In this chapter, we put into perspective the critiques presented in this book. In the course of reviewing the chapter drafts, we reached two conclusions with regard to what they conveyed collectively. First, the record of African governments' responses to the HIV/AIDS pandemic displays a pattern of incidental as opposed to transformational leadership. There is a preponderance of reactions to developments in the spread of the disease and in the means of curtailing it amongst heads of state and national executives, which we view as illustrations of incidental leadership. There is less evidence of transformational leadership; that is, interventions by leaders to ensure consistency over time in decision-making, in setting and revising priorities and, as necessary, in changing or transforming society. Second, much of the public criticism of African governments' efforts to curb HIV and AIDS reflects people's experience and perceptions of a denial of citizenship. In this instance, borrowing from Jacques Derrida (1997), we argue that any attempt on the part of the government to propose a policy or implement it in a way detrimental to the well-being of its people, especially on the matter of HIV/AIDS, redefines the citizen (*cives*) as an enemy (*inimicus/hostis*).

Our argument hinges on discussion of two overlapping issues. One is the concept of the state and its articulation in Africa in relation to government's responses to the HIV/AIDS pandemic. The other is the rhetoric on HIV/AIDS voiced by Africa's heads of state since the 1980s. We provide the basis for discussion of these issues in the following section. Thereafter, we discuss the variations within and between African government's responses since the 1980s to show how and why African governments have been and continue to be targets for criticism. We then place the discussion within the context of African governments' collective record as expressed in the African Union's (AU) deliberations on HIV/AIDS. Our purpose here is to illustrate our argument with regard to incidental and transformational leadership. Our rationale is that the AU represents the collective voice of the vast majority of African governments and through joint declarations of heads of state and ministers it has regularly proclaimed their common cause, principles and strategies with regard to HIV/AIDS. Therefore, the AU has set the standards of leadership by which the heads of state and ministers have pronounced they should be judged.

HIV/AIDS and the state

The concept of the state refers to an institution that is responsible for the management of a geo-political space and allocation of resources to meet defined societal needs. The management and provision of public health services has become one responsibility of the state throughout Africa. However, there are good reasons to doubt African states' commitment to that responsibility.

In the first instance, our doubt is based on wide-ranging critiques of African states during the latter half of the twentieth century. We refer here to the vast literature on the challenges of the transition from colonialism to political independence, the wars in Africa, the history of foreign aid and externally driven reshaping of states represented, for example, by structural adjustment programmes. In the field of public health, our doubts stem from indications of resurgences of previously contained diseases such as measles and polio, shortages of doctors and nurses in many countries (WHO 2006a, 2006c) and, in relation to HIV/AIDS, evidence of the need for substantive redesign of health services (Beck et al. 2006).

Second, any discussion about African states' capacities and capabilities invokes the notion of citizenship; specifically, a national government's control or lack thereof over a territorial space and its inhabitants, coupled with a contractual commitment to enhance the welfare of those inhabitants and the environment in which they live. The limits of this commitment continue to be contested around the globe, as reflected in public debates about the extent of welfare services that governments can and should support in a rapidly changing world. However, in an age of Internet communications, extensive migrancy and growing national populations in the diaspora, Africans have become very aware of the broader limits of government commitment in democratic, developed countries compared to the more narrow limits found throughout Africa. A foreigner, for instance, can receive free medical care in a public hospital in Britain and some Scandinavian countries and, elsewhere in Europe, medical attention prior to requests for payment. In stark contrast, South African citizens who do not possess identity documents are frequently denied access to public health and social services in their own country. Furthermore, individuals who have health insurance are fortunate when they find hospitals that do not demand proof of capability to pay before receiving treatment. Africans who visit or work in African countries other than their own, know that medical services are assured only if they can pay for them.

Third, citizens' rights to healthcare have been tempered by the promotion of private healthcare services throughout the world, which serve those who are formally employed and who have recourse to medical insurance schemes. Some countries, such as Nigeria, have implemented national health insurance schemes (Ogundiran, Fatumbi and Costantinos 2006: 220) but these are rare in Africa. Instead, secular and religious non-governmental organisations (NGOs) have been at the forefront of efforts to improve all people's access to public health services.

It is this history and context which lends weight to judgements of African states such as the following: 'Public health budgets are no longer seen as productive investment for human development and economic growth but an unnecessary financial burden on governments which should be avoided' (Poku and Whiteside 2004: 1).

Assessing explanations of African governments' responses to HIV/AIDS

When he was Secretary-General of the United Nations, Kofi Annan asserted: 'Our response was . . . shockingly late and shamefully ill-resourced and donors are not providing anything like the amount of aid needed to halt the pandemic' (UN 2004: 9; see also UNAIDS 2008: 8–10).

A slow or delayed response of political authorities and a lack of resources have become axioms in the recorded history of HIV/AIDS in Africa. We question this judgement, as a first step to disentangling criticisms about African governments' responses to HIV/AIDS. The criticisms revolve not only around expectations that political authorities should and can lead interventions on HIV/AIDS. They also refer to the grounds on which strategic decisions are made and, in particular, to the moral implications of decisions about who is affected, who should be assisted and why. Government decisions were and still are 'life-and-death' decisions; people can quickly discern the probable consequences for themselves and others. Inevitably such consideration leads to questioning the rationality of the decisions and, ultimately, whether Africa's political leaders are doing right or wrong regarding their citizens.

Stated more formally, authority and subject argue in a context of partial knowledge about the biochemical nature of the disease, the psycho-social and socio-economic effects, the primacy of sexual transmission of the virus in Africa, the different means to make sense of HIV and AIDS and about the moral options which underpin use of that knowledge. Objective, technical information is only one (and not necessarily the most important) basis for debate in this context.[1] Criticism of the leadership displayed by African governments is wide ranging and covers past, present and future. The accusation of a 'slow' or 'delayed response', for example, is an historical judgement while pleas of 'lack of resources' refer to the present. Both prefigure concern about the quality of leadership, popularly expressed in terms of the presence or absence of political will. Political will prefigures assessments about the rightness and wrongness of a government's actions, which, as we illustrate later, can change rapidly.[2] In other words, any assessment of government responses has to consider many different factors; thus our caution about accepting 'slow response' judgements.

Early efforts to describe the disease highlighted the limited knowledge about HIV/AIDS. It came to public and government attention in Africa shortly after warnings were voiced in the United States in the late 1970s and indications that the virus was to be found more in homosexual populations and less in heterosexual populations (Altman 1986; Preda 2005: 67–112; Illiffe 2006: 1–32). Subsequently, human sexuality became a foundation for categorising patterns in the spread of HIV. North America, Latin America, Western Europe and Australasia geographically demarcated a concentration of HIV prevalence amongst the homosexual population. East, Central and Southern Africa and the Caribbean were the locations where HIV was prevalent in the heterosexual population. North Africa, Asia, Eastern Europe and the Pacific were areas where there was inadequate information to make a classification (Siedel and Vidal 1997: 61; Hankin et al. 2006).

Sexual disposition was an imperfect means to guide an understanding of HIV/AIDS. Coupled with indications of significant rates of HIV transmission via injections (recipients of blood transfusions; people who injected drugs for recreational purposes), it allowed for interpretations of HIV infection as a consequence of deviant behaviour. This tagging has spawned equally prejudicial explanations about African governments' responses to HIV/AIDS, which continue to confound debates. Xolela Mangcu (2008: 50), for example, argues that the South African government of the apartheid era (1961–94) categorised AIDS as a 'gay disease', inferring that the government did not view the disease as a significant public health threat because of inherent prejudice (homosexual intercourse was illegal at the time) and a belief that homosexuality was not common in the country's population. There certainly was prejudice of this nature within government circles but it was not confined to that agency alone. It was prevalent throughout society and elsewhere in the world throughout the 1980s (Lawson 2008).[3] Prejudice, coupled with fear, became very convoluted as Lawson (2008: 21–47) illustrates; for example, evidence of a growing epidemic amongst the heterosexual population and amongst migrant workers in the mid-1980s was rebuffed by the National Union of Mineworkers for being racist by supposedly suggesting that 'black' people were sexually promiscuous. Lawson infers that an effect was a 'slow' response by the government but she also reveals factors that, we contend, contradict that inference. We refer here to the fact that debates about HIV/AIDS in the 1980s (throughout the world, not only in South Africa) were shaped by very limited knowledge of the disease and, as importantly, by the limitations of the knowledge that was being gained.

On the one hand, clinical and public information at the time was derived largely from the effects and experiences of HIV and AIDS in the gay community of the United States and amongst injecting drug users; in short, the threat seemed limited to particular sub-populations. The initial response and relative success in curtailing the spread of the virus amongst the gay population in the United States came from those affected, not from the intervention of the government or international health agencies. On the other hand, clinical and research evidence highlighted general symptoms of the disease, not a thorough understanding of the causes and possible means to cure or contain it. We refer here to the evidence of a rapid spread of the disease through sexual intercourse and to the seemingly elusive nature of the virus, which frustrated efforts to develop a vaccine and other efficacious medicines.[4] In other words, governments were struggling with the available evidence to find a sound basis on which to make decisions, not only with regard to the level and scale of intervention required but also how to intervene in the absence of an obvious medical answer.

HIV/AIDS came to public attention in Africa as a potentially significant threat in the early to mid-1980s. In Nigeria, for example, the first infection is said to have been reported in April 1986 and, in the same year, the Ministry of Health established a special task team to investigate (Ogundiran, Fatumbi and Costantinos 2006: 221). Ogundiran, Fatumbi and Costantinos (224) assert that, subsequently, the 'level of response in this period was very low' in view of the emphasis on health education and HIV prevention. Most interventions were driven by external agencies and the first prevalence surveys were commissioned in 1991, followed by others in 1993. The results of these surveys suggested that prevalence rates had risen from 2% of the population to 10%. However, the Nigerian government began to seek clarity about the problem in much the same fashion as other governments: its second survey was conducted relatively rapidly after the first to enable assessment of the scale of the problem.

Likewise, in South Africa, the Medical Research Council began to sponsor research in 1982-3 at the time when the first HIV case was formally reported.[5] Public awareness increased throughout the 1980s, as did research and official concern, though this was constrained by the civil unrest during that time. There was a remarkable joint effort by government officials and those of the African National Congress (ANC), including those in exile, to put HIV/AIDS high on the political agenda in 1990-1. Furthermore, during the tense period (1992-4) of political negotiations, the National AIDS Committee of South Africa (NACOSA) was created. Consequently, when a political democracy was established in 1994, South Africa had a plan to confront the disease (Schneider 1998; Stein and Zwi 1990).

Similar processes occurred elsewhere (Beck et al. 2006). The timing varied for each country during the 1980s but governments responded and went on to elaborate those responses as medical and public knowledge increased in the 1990s. In other words, to criticise governments for a 'slow' response is problematic because such criticism discounts the lack of knowledge about the disease at the time and the necessary steps taken to establish structures and means to assess the threat and to devise strategic reactions.

We suggest it is more useful to recognise that the criticism is really directed at the effectiveness of government responses. However, assessments of effectiveness are fraught with complications. The terms of reference, or more colloquially, the playing field and the goal posts, are frequently shifting. There are two factors complicating debates about the effectiveness of governments' responses. First, the principal means to measure effectiveness, HIV prevalence and mortality rates, are not as useful as they appear to be.[6] Effectiveness is measured over time, the key factor being whether there is a discernable rise or decline in the rates subsequent to interventions. This exercise can be useful for an overview but rates and trends by themselves do not show any link to interventions. Second, the context emphasises a search for answers to questions about what needs to be done now, what needs to be tested to check if it works, what policies, strategies and plans should be devised in relation to current conditions and whether existing interventions are being implemented appropriately to achieve good effects. To illustrate these complications, we refer to Senegal and South Africa as representing two extremes of African governments' interpretation of partial knowledge about HIV/AIDS.

Senegal is an African country where the government prevented an HIV/AIDS epidemic: prevalence rates have not risen above 1% (Simms, Sow and Sy 2006: 228–39). References to Senegal generally contain the implicit argument that the success has been achieved despite it being poor, lacking resources and having marked socio-economic inequalities between the rich and the poor and between men and women (Meda et al. 1999; Putzel 2003; Simms, Sow and Sy 2006; Willems 2009) and, explicitly, that Senegal's success is due to sound leadership: 'Political leadership and conservative sexual mores were both important in the fight against HIV, together with Senegal's long tradition of taking a pragmatic and participatory approach to primary prevention' (Simms, Sow and Sy 2006: 228).

In contrast, South Africa has achieved notoriety in and beyond Africa for what is popularly known as 'Mbeki's denialism'. This refers to the strategies and policies of the national government under the presidency of Thabo Mbeki from 1998 to 2008. Those years witnessed many disputes between the government and civil society as the country's HIV prevalence rose rapidly, leading to estimations that AIDS was becoming the principal contributor to mortality in South Africa. Statistical calculations estimate that HIV prevalence rose from less than 1% in 1990 to 25% (approximately four million individuals) in 2001 (Dorrington, Bradshaw and Budlender 2002). Estimates since then indicate that the general prevalence has stayed between 20 and 30%, with variations according to age, gender and location (Department of Health 2005; HSRC 2009).

One feature of Mbeki's denialism was his manipulation of the sexual classification of HIV/AIDS to promote a strategy that restricted public access to antiretroviral (ARV) treatment, favoured nutritional support for those infected and emphasised socio-economic development initiatives. Mbeki did not support this alternative strategy on its own merits but through reviving the prejudices and doubts of the 1980s about the disease. In brief, he argued that concerns about the rising levels of heterosexual HIV infection in Africa disguised racist explanations (the intimation that 'black' people were sexually promiscuous); that international planning discourse served Western ideological interests; and that medical science was ignoring the possibility of AIDS being a function of poverty rather than the HI virus.[7] Chapters 4, 5 and 10 in this volume discuss these contests in detail and Chapters 8 and 9 include pertinent background discussion (see also Brink 2000; Butler 2005; Goldacre 2009; Grundlingh 2001; Quinlan and Willan 2004; Weinel 2005; Willan 2004).

Senegal and South Africa represent extremes in Africa in several ways: divergent perspectives on the sexual dynamics of HIV transmission; success and failure to control a national epidemic; systematic and fractured strategies. They exemplify the difference between transformational and incidental leadership; specifically, the contrast among systemic and evidence and results-oriented interventions to initiate changes in society, on the one hand and, on the other, reactive, problem-focused interventions. We elaborate on these points below.

In Senegal, the first HIV case was reported in 1986. Senegalese clinical scientists had previously worked to discover a strain of the virus and convinced the then president, Mr Abdou Diouf, of the threat it posed (Meda et al. 1999; Putzel 2003). Consequently, in 1988, the Multi-disciplinary National Committee for the Prevention of AIDS was formed to implement the country's first HIV/AIDS campaign. The campaign focused on prevention of inadvertent transmission of the virus via blood transfusions through rigorous screening of all blood donations; prevention of sexual transmission of the virus through an education and awareness campaign promoting responsible and safe sex, including provision of condoms; widespread screening and treatment of sexually transmitted infections; and focused interventions for categories of people considered to have a high risk of sexual exposure to HIV (Willems 2009).[8] In 1992, the country's Department of Education introduced a comprehensive HIV module in all schools. Furthermore, by 1995, the government and the religious authorities, predominantly Muslim clerics, had reached agreement on combined programmes that included endorsement of traditional social and sexual norms alongside promotion of condom use and incorporation of AIDS education and tolerance in religious teachings (Putzel 2003; Willems 2009).

In South Africa, there was the remarkable development of NACOSA and an HIV/AIDS intervention plan to guide the new government after 1994. However, that was abandoned within three years as the government cultivated an alternative approach. Thereafter, the government's AIDS initiatives were marked by controversy. Shifts in the loci of authority were a marked feature of disputes between the government and civil organisations. Government disputes with scientists, for example, led to the replacement of the board of the Medicines Control Council, which is the arbiter for decisions on what medicines are approved and the protocols for their use. The message was that the council's decision-making was to be subordinate to the political stance of the government. Mr Mbeki created a presidential advisory body that included 'HIV dissident' scientists (those who questioned the relationship between HIV and AIDS) as well as 'mainstream' senior scientists. Consequently, this initiative failed because there was no agreement between the two sets of scientists. The South African National AIDS Council (SANAC) was overshadowed by the Treatment Action Campaign (TAC), an NGO that advocated stridently for the government to implement ARV programmes, and the judiciary, which eventually compelled the government to do so. SANAC's principal role, to co-ordinate government and non-government initiatives, was also eclipsed by promotion of co-ordinated planning and action by the 'social cluster' ministries (health, education and social development) at national and provincial levels of government according, ironically, to the constitutionally sanctioned principle of co-operative governance.

In summary, how, as opposed to when, governments responded to HIV/AIDS is the source of debate about the effectiveness of those responses. This issue also has its own axiom. Political will, its presence or absence, is a popular way of summarising governments' actions and the quality of leadership. It became part of the lexicon of HIV/AIDS in the 1990s as a result of the concerted efforts of the Ugandan government and, beyond Africa, Thailand's government, to prevent the spread of the virus in their countries. Those efforts were associated with the marked decrease in national HIV prevalence in Uganda and in Thailand – national rates of 4.1% and 1.5% respectively (Hankin et al. 2006: 23, 30).

Botswana has also become an exemplar in Africa following the government-led introduction of a comprehensive treatment strategy in 2001 in the face of evidence indicating a massive HIV epidemic: 39% of 15–49-year-olds reported HIV-positive in 2000 and 285 000 total were infected in a population of 1.6 million (Lush, Darkoh and Ramotlhwa 2006: 181, 184, 192). The Botswana government's strategy has included the provision of ARVs to all in need, collaboration with NGOs and international health agencies and pharmaceutical companies and, since 2006, extensive expansion of health facilities coupled with monetary incentives to attract medical staff from elsewhere in Africa and beyond.

Following improvements in medical therapies, knowledge that ARVs could turn HIV infection from being a death sentence into a chronic illness introduced a new basis for assessing political will. This basis has four components: the provision of ARV medicines; the ease of access to the medicines for those in need; the support provided to patients to maintain treatment regimes; and the extent to which interventions confront the psycho-social and socio-economic effects of the disease on families. To date, the patchy record of governments' programmes on one or more of these components fuels public doubt about the political will of their leaders.

No country in Africa is known to provide ARV medicines to all those in need. A perennial refrain of international and local agencies is the gap between the numbers who are on treatment and those who should be (WHO 2008). Access to treatment is constrained throughout Africa; all countries have sparse networks of health service facilities. The facilities are concentrated in the towns and cities and, in rural areas they are at least an hour and up to a day's travel for the vast majority of residents (Beck et al. 2006). Support services across Africa are often rudimentary and, in the absence of government facilities, provided largely by NGOs and community initiatives. Support services are limited as they require a range of interventions, such as professional review and adjustment of individual treatment regimes, counselling, nutritional guidance, home-based care programmes and orphan care (Bärngihausen, Bloom and Humair 2007; Chen et al. 2004; Hanefeld and Musheke 2009; Huicho et al. 2008).

These limitations underlie other problems. The procurement and supply of medicines was a significant problem throughout the continent in the early 2000s. These years were marked by advocacy, legal contests and negotiations over the use of branded and generic medicines, for example, and quality control of new medicines (Wilson, Cohen-Kohler and Whiteside 2008). Some countries have committed to creating free public ARV programmes; others require some payment (HEARD 2009). A minority of every national population, local elites and people in formal employment whose employers subscribe to health insurance schemes can access well-resourced private health services (HEARD 2009). The majority continue to rely on under-resourced and understaffed public health services.[9]

Nonetheless, people can assess the effectiveness of government interventions on the basis of observable conditions, such as the availability of services; the quality of counselling; the extent of government social support structures, such as grants and home-based care programmes and, of course, people recovering their health. This is in marked contrast to the days when the emphasis was on preventing HIV transmission. Education and awareness campaigns, condom distribution programmes and exhortations to people to change their sexual behaviour were necessary and the message could be heard and felt. However, the effects were not visible nor were they convincingly demonstrated in graphic representations of changes in prevalence and mortality rates.[10]

Our point is that the introduction of ARVs changed the terms of reference for assessing government actions. In turn, a principal measure of a government's political will has become its capability to implement programmes that demonstrate consistency in the provision of treatment and continuity of care.[11] Key criteria are how governments harness and deploy existing resources, whether and how they develop capacity (bearing in mind the massive financial support from international agencies) and what use they make of new knowledge; in sum, whether they demonstrate the capability to manage resources. Governments fuel public scepticism about their commitments and capabilities when they ignore these criteria. Such scepticism is expressed in many ways. For instance, government officials regularly get caught on the wrong foot when they use statistics that reveal apparent decreases in HIV prevalence or mortality rates to suggest government commitment and capability. One example of this was at a conference in Addis Ababa in 2007 convened to review the results of a large social science research programme that had been supported by the Swedish International Development Cooperation Agency (SIDA). Scientists from Burkina Faso and Kenya took to task the presentations by representatives of their respective countries' National AIDS Councils (NACs). The NAC representatives made the mistake of trying to convince the audience that HIV prevalence in the two countries was decreasing due to government interventions. Criticism was vocal and heated. It included standard critiques, such as the limited time frames used in the analyses and the questionable validity of the estimates.[12] The main criticism was incredulity at the NAC representatives' failure to acknowledge the import of the large body of research presented at the conference. In essence, this research revealed the challenges of containing the spread of the disease in localities and different sub-populations and the lost opportunities for governments to use research evidence and to support the multitude of initiatives within communities.

Another significant source of public scepticism is growing awareness of the different levels of achievement across Africa. Thirty years into the pandemic, there are now testimonies about how and where epidemics have and have not been contained. There is a small yet expanding record of assessments of interventions and of changes in policies and practice (Beck et al. 2006; Campbell 2003; Guillespie 2006; Pisani 2008). Illustration is provided in this book in Chapter 4. There are still gaps in the information but enough knowledge for the public to pose critical questions: How and why are some countries 'succeeding' while others are not? What can be learned from other countries? Are African governments learning from each other? These questions also cast doubt on the common argument that a lack of resources accounts for limitations of national programmes. There is no denying the need for very large sums of money as well as substantial investment in human resources and infrastructure. However, the argument is becoming increasingly weak in view of successes not being restricted to countries that are wealthier than others. There have been and still are large flows of international funding. There is now a vast body of research information and experience to inform the design and operation of interventions. There are also longstanding organisational principles and means for identifying, conserving and improving the use of resources (for example, decentralisation; primary health care; co-ordination and integration) (Bolland and Wilson 1994; Mills et al. 1990; UNAIDS 2004, 2005; Walt et al. 2008; WHO 2003, 2008).[13]

These considerations direct attention to whether African governments are confronting HIV/AIDS systematically. Judgements depend as much on governments being seen to be systematic as on the actual results of national strategies. The success of some countries in containing the spread of HIV shows what can be done. In short, the question is, are governments going forward? A number of criteria as outlined above are being used to give answers. The measures are imprecise but apposite in a context of partial knowledge; for instance, comparisons of different countries providing some benchmarks for progress. Uganda is a country seen to have contained a large epidemic. Botswana is a country with a large epidemic but the government is seen to be acting decisively and systematically. The governments of Tanzania and Kenya, countries with smaller epidemics, are gaining in standing for the same reasons. In contrast, the Swaziland government is notorious for consistently failing to confront HIV/AIDS systematically despite the best efforts of NGOs and the National Emergency Response Committee on HIV/AIDS (equivalent to a NAC) (Whiteside, Whalley and Naysmith 2007).

There is little evidence, however, of African governments learning from each other and providing mutual support. Seemingly, as we outlined earlier, they are always one or more steps behind the changes in the terms of reference for policy debates. Furthermore, past achievements count for little if a government stumbles in developing and refining its interventions in line with globally recognised strategies and also in relation to foreseeable future demands. In other words, governments can and do 'lose the plot' as we indicated in the case of South Africa during the Mbeki era. Likewise, there is now doubt about Uganda's momentum. Uganda won renown for effective interventions through promotion of its locally conceived ABC (Abstain, Be Faithful, Condomise) and 'zero-grazing' (promotion of monogamous relationships) programmes. However, there is doubt about the efficacy of the government's efforts since the mid-2000s in view of its endorsement of sexual abstinence campaigns supported financially by American government funding and backed by some Christian groups. More recently, in 2010, the national government's overt condemnation of homosexuality contradicts the emphasis on human rights in the design of interventions and the people-centred strategy to improve healthcare services endorsed by the World Health Organization (WHO 2008).[14]

Leaving aside, for the moment, moral and rights criteria, doubts about the quality of leadership are either exacerbated or dispelled according to governments' responses to the demands of developing ARV programmes and continuity of care. In due course, governments will need to show the effectiveness of treatment interventions by using empirical measures, such as the number of people on treatment in relation to demand and the number of patients who have recovered their health in relation to numbers of deaths.

We have discussed the prisms through which people discern ambivalence on the part of African governments to care for their citizens: in essence, how they react to new knowledge of the disease, to new technologies and, thereafter, to the inevitable changes to the terms for debates on strategy and policy. This ambivalence can be measured in terms of a government's commitment (or lack thereof) to go forward in ways that are beneficial for its citizens. We elaborate on these points in the next section.

Assessing African governments' commitment to curtailing the HIV/AIDS pandemic

Our focus here is on African governments collectively and, for this purpose, we refer to the AU's decisions and actions on HIV/AIDS. We outline the historical record of the AU's deliberations on HIV/AIDS to illustrate the tenor of the rhetoric. Thereafter, we assess its record, arguing that the perennial proclamations of concern and commitment to the welfare of Africa's inhabitants belie the quality of executive leadership in Africa.

As a starting point, we draw on Benedict Anderson's treatise on the temporality of a nation state's conduct, expressed succinctly here: 'if nations can, at least hypothetically, be Wrong, this wrongness is temporal, and is always set against a transcendental Right and Good' (1998: 360). In other words, critical assessments of a government (or governments) should not ignore a larger yet subliminal reference point that invariably frames an analysis. This is the place of government policies and strategies, actions and events, and their effects on people, within the broader history of a nation state. Subjects of an assessment include not only the living but also, and often tacitly, the dead and the unborn and not only the present, but also the past and future welfare of the nation (360–4). Accordingly, critiques that highlight faults in a government at a particular moment in history do not derive their authority only from evidence of the moment. They also rely on benchmarks consisting of morals, principles and societal goals; in essence, a purpose proclaimed by a government and society at large that expresses (and is expressed in diverse ways) a desired condition of well-being for all.

Anderson's commentary provides a useful foundation for assessing African governments' commitment to curtailing the HIV/AIDS pandemic. Any assessment is, at root, a consideration of whether, where and how a government is right or wrong in its deliberations and actions. This book makes this consideration overt via the focus on the apparent ambivalence of African governments to HIV/AIDS. However, Anderson's caveat about the temporality of 'wrongness' is apt. It reminds us that the record of African governments' commitment is not uniformly 'bad' and that any consideration of ambivalence is about discerning resonances as well as dissonances within and between what governments say and what they do. With these points in mind, we outline first the AU's declarations on HIV/AIDS and then present a critique.

The AU is a remodelled version (in July 2002) of the Organisation of African Unity (OAU) (Adebajo, Adedeji and Landsberg 2007: 198). It is an initiative to promote co-operation among 54 independent member states on the African continent.[15] Currently, the AU includes all African countries except Morocco. Its core mandate is to decide on policy of common interest to the members. The organs of the AU include heads of government, ministers and the nascent Pan African Parliament (198). It is known to the public largely by the summits it organises and the declarations it issues which, in principle, are binding on all members. For the purposes of our critique, we discuss the AU declarations on HIV/AIDS under four time periods: 1991-4, 1995-2000, 2001-5 and 2006 to the present.[16] The periods approximate different moments of development in the AU's deliberations.

1991-4

The OAU discussed the issue of HIV/AIDS in Abuja in 1991 at a meeting of heads of state and governments and issued its first decisions and declaration on the matter. Consistent with the times, the declaration viewed HIV/AIDS primarily as an additional, major public health threat as is indicated in the following quote: 'We feel concerned of the foreseeable trend in the health crisis due to:

- Uncontrolled AIDS pandemic
- Resurfacing with increased frequency of malaria, cholera, plague, meningitis and yellow fever
- Insufficient organisation of local communities for their full participation in health and development' (OAU 1991: AHG/Decl. 3, 4).

The declaration committed all the heads of governments to 'strengthen national health systems', 'to resolve the health crisis' through a range of interventions, including: 'inter-African co-operation in the field of health' (emphasising 'reinforcement' of community health organisations); 'intensifying their [communities'] current co-operation with governments (emphasising people-centred, community-oriented policies, strategies and action plans); 'encouraging exchange of experiences and health information between countries' and 'inter-country co-operation' as well as what are now common strategies, such as a multisectoral approach and focused HIV/AIDS prevention interventions. The declaration ended with an imperative to national health ministers to report back on their implementation of the declaration to the Secretary-General of the OAU by 1995.

A year later the OAU issued a second set of decisions and declarations on HIV/AIDS from an assembly of heads of state held in Dakar, Senegal (OAU 1992: AHG/Decl. 1. XXVIII). This document conveyed greater concern (for example, 'by the year 2000, it is estimated 20 million Africans will be HIV positive causing 1 million deaths annually'; 'We must emphasize the gravity and urgency of the epidemic') and included a commitment to 'An Agenda for Action'. The first part of this document is a collective identification with the threat of HIV/AIDS. The second part expresses a commitment (denoted below as C) to collective action, corresponding with six stated targets (denoted below as T):

- (C1) 'by giving our fullest political commitment to mobilizing society as a whole for the fight';
- (T1) 'by the end of 1992, each one of us will be publicly recognized as the leader of the fight against AIDS in one's own country';

- (C2) 'by stepping up to prevent sexual transmission of HIV';
- (T2) 'by mid 1993, all of us will have ensured that 100% of our country's adults, including young adults, know how HIV is transmitted and how they can protect themselves and others from infections';
- (C3) 'by planning for the care of people with HIV infection and AIDS and the support of their families and survivors';
- (T3) 'by mid 1993, we will have adopted a national AIDS care plan, including essential drugs for HIV-related illness, and a plan for the family of community-based care and support of AIDS survivors, including orphans';
- (C4) 'by supporting appropriate and relevant AIDS research';
- (T4) 'by the end of 1993, we will have endorsed a National Plan of Action for the Promotion and Coordination of AIDS Research in our countries including an operational ethical code in AIDS Research';
- (C5) 'by using our leadership position to ensure that all sectors of society work together to tackle the AIDS epidemic';
- (T5) 'by the end of 1993, we will have ensured that every sector has worked out a plan, and allocated funds to it that takes into account the sectoral implications and consequences of AIDS, and will have established an effective high-level mechanism for the multi-sectoral coordination of the planned activities';
- (C6) 'we must make AIDS a top priority for external resource allocation so that our continent benefits from maximum international cooperation and solidarity in overcoming the epidemic and its impact';
- (T6) 'by the end of 1994, we will have collaborated in and produced a consolidated Plan of Action for Africa to attract the financing needed for controlling AIDS and containing the epidemic's consequences, and will begin to promote this Plan of Action' (OAU 1992: AHG/Decl. 1. XXVIII).

The third part includes an additional 'Resolution on AIDS and Africa: An Agenda for Action' (OAU 1992: AHG/Res. 216) which reiterates the concern and commitment; for example, with recommendations emphasising that 'no effort be spared', directives to national ministers of health to develop comprehensive action plans and requests for collaboration with international agencies. The next two declarations indicate a commitment to progressive and focused interventions by the member states. The 1994 declaration, for example, encouraged the heads of state to:

- create national policy frameworks;
- protect young people from HIV;
- promote and support applied research; and
- make substantial budgetary provisions for prevention programmes (OAU 1994: AHG/Decl. 1).

It also included an emphatic statement: 'We commit ourselves to follow closely the implementation of this declaration'.

In sum, the declarations suggest substantive commitment by the continent's political leadership, expressed in terms of personal and collective concern ('our continent'; 'our people'), will-power ('we commit ourselves') and authority ('We, the heads of States'). However, there was ambiguity in the rhetoric, notably in the terminology of 'we' and in statements of how the commitment was to be exercised (see Billig 1991, 1996). It was contradicted by directives for each state to act independently in terms of translating the declarations into practical actions. The OAU's deliberations were also overshadowed by political conflicts on the continent. For instance, the OAU chairperson for 1992–3, Ibrahim Babangida, the president of Nigeria, left Dakar to face political unrest at home following his cancellation of the country's general elections in 1993 and subsequently, his gradual loss of domestic political authority. Liberia, the Democratic Republic of Congo, Angola, Ethiopia, Eritrea and Somalia were enmeshed in civil wars and South Africa was engaged in political negotiations to end apartheid.

1995–2000

The mid-1990s initially marked a contrast to the early 1990s in terms of the opportunities for the OAU to capitalise on the sound policy injunctions contained in preceding declarations. In South Africa, for example, the remarkable process of the negotiated and participatory transition to democracy was reflected in the existence of a national plan to confront HIV/AIDS that had been formulated collaboratively through discussions since 1991 by political leaders and health professionals from opposing sides. Furthermore, the issue of HIV/AIDS was championed by President Nelson Mandela in and beyond South Africa. Nigeria had returned to civil rule under its president, Olusegun Obasanjo, and the latter overtly championed initiatives, at home and across the continent, to confront the HIV pandemic. A number of countries were emerging from civil strife (Liberia; the Democratic Republic of Congo and Angola). Zimbabwe had yet to descend into political turmoil.

The OAU's declaration of 1995, emanating from a meeting held in Addis Ababa, was subtly different to the instructive tenor of the previous declarations and contained more reflective injunctions. HIV/AIDS was included in a 'plan of action' that focused on promoting maternal and child health and welfare and the emphasis was on encouraging appropriate interventions (OAU 1995: AHG/Decl. 1-2).

However, for the most part, the decisions and declarations during this period reveal no substantive development on those in the preceding documents; indeed, the texts convey a focus on problems rather than solutions. In the 1996 declarations of a meeting held in Yaoundé (OAU 1996: Decl. 1-4), the 'resolution on HIV/AIDS' (AHG/Res. 247) focused on concerns about the slow implementation of the HIV/AIDS agenda, fears that the pandemic might negate the social and economic gains of some African countries and the need to appeal to donor agencies for support, alongside affirmations about dedication to combat the disease and for regular reporting of actions to the OAU secretariat.

The 1997 health-related declaration from a meeting in Harare (OAU 1997: AHG/Decl. 1-4) focused on malaria prevention and control. The 1998 declaration from a session held in Ouagadougou, Burkina Faso emphasised a WHO 'Roll Back Malaria' initiative in Africa but included affirmation of the Dakar and Tunis declarations as well as support for a proposed 'Solidarity Fund to help treatment of patients from Africa' (OAU 1998: AHG/Decl. 124, 125).

2001–5

The OAU/AU's deliberations in the early years of this decade have been marked by reaffirmations of the need for comprehensive interventions, including international support, on major diseases in Africa in view of their co-presence and their threat to social and economic order.[17] A much-cited report was that of the 'Special Summit on HIV/AIDS, TB and Other Related Infectious Diseases', hosted by the then Nigerian president, Olusegun Obasanjo, in Abuja in 2001 (OAU 2001a). It reiterated concerns and commitments expressed in previous OAU declarations (for example, 'We consider AIDS as a State of Emergency in the continent'; 'We commit ourselves to take personal responsibility and leadership for the activities of National AIDS Commissions/Councils'). It is credited in subsequent decisions and declarations of the AU with promoting continent-wide co-ordination of efforts and international partnerships.[18] However, the report from the meeting in Lome, Togo in 2000 actually emphasises in more detail the importance and need for co-ordination and partnerships (OAU 2000: AHG/Decl. 3). The import of the Abuja 2001 meeting really lies in the fact that it was championed by Olusegun Obasanjo and, as we will discuss shortly, is an initiative that has been repeated and has provided impetus for AU deliberations on HIV/AIDS throughout this decade. Furthermore, the Abuja meeting was the occasion at which an advocacy group, AIDS Watch Africa, was formed. It consisted of the heads of state from Botswana, Ethiopia, Kenya, Mali, Nigeria, Rwanda, South Africa and Uganda, with Obasanjo co-ordinating the group (AWA 2006).[19]

Decisions of a 2001 meeting in Lusaka, Zambia affirmed the Abuja declaration (OAU 2001b: AHG/Decl. 2). Decisions from a 2003 meeting in Maputo, Mozambique, reflected key components of the international HIV/AIDS agenda and also reiterated many elements of preceding declarations (AU 2003: Decl. 6). The report of a meeting in 2005, again in Abuja, was consistent with the preceding declarations and decisions of this decade but emphasised the importance of international support, co-ordination and partnerships alongside Africa's inability to finance HIV/AIDS interventions alone (AU 2005: Decl. 55).

2006 to the present

The mid-decade is notable for a second Abuja summit held in 2006. The focus was on promoting universal access for people in Africa to HIV/AIDS and TB treatment and to sexual and reproductive health services (AU 2006a, 2006b). The decisions and declarations from this summit contain a long list of 'Guiding Principles To Which Africa Will Adhere' for national HIV/AIDS interventions (AU 2006a: 4).[20] They also defined 'Targets To Be Met by 2010':

- Reduce HIV prevalence in young people between 15 and 24 years, by at least 25% in ALL African countries;
- protect and support in 2010, 5 million children orphaned by AIDS and ensure that 80% of orphans and vulnerable children have access to basic services;
- at least 80% of pregnant women have access to prevention of mother-to-child transmission (PMTCT) and treatment for HIV-positive women and children;
- at least 80% of those in need, particularly children, have access to HIV/AIDS treatment, especially antiretroviral, as well as care and support (AU 2006a: 5).

The document also committed heads of state to developing and refining national plans as necessary to achieve the targets, including specification of revised interim and final targets by December 2006. The rhetoric was unambiguous; for example:

- Member States of the African Union will intensify the fight against HIV/AIDS and achieve other internationally agreed goals on health (AU 2006a: 5);
- since progress towards these bold collective goals can only be assured through decisive action at the country level, we commit to . . .;

- specifically, We African Heads of State and Government undertake to: Provide bold and resolute leadership in spearheading efforts in all countries to combat HIV/AIDS, TB and Malaria; Implement, in all countries, the commitments adopted at the Special Summit in Abuja, Nigeria in 2006; Provide bold and resolute leadership in spearheading efforts in all countries to combat HIV/AIDS, TB and Malaria (and six other related and equally emphatic actions) (AU 2006a: 6).

Since then, however, AU decisions and declarations on HIV/AIDS have been relatively brief and intermittent. References are made, often as reminders ('recalling . . .'), primarily to the 2001 and 2006 Abuja declarations but also to earlier declarations. The texts consist largely of text copied or paraphrased from previous declarations. Only three of the nine AU general sessions since 2006 mention HIV/AIDS.[21] The meeting in Banjul in 2006 is noteworthy for emphasising the need for the 'harmonization' of approaches (AU 2006d: Decl. 116).[22] A meeting in Sharm-el Sheikh, Egypt, in 2008 acknowledged a progress report on the Abuja 2006 declaration (AU 2008: Decl. 194).[23] A meeting of the AU executive council held in Kampala, Uganda in July 2010 recommended a proposal from Senegal for 'A partnership for elimination of mother to child transmission of HIV in Africa' (AU 2010: Ex.cl/Decl. 584). In summary, the high points of the AU's deliberations on HIV/AIDS this decade have been the Abuja declarations and a collective position on HIV/AIDS that is in alignment with the agenda of international health agencies.

Leadership: What kind of leadership?
The AU's deliberations for the last nineteen years are remarkable for revealing very few moments of collective action on overtly moral grounds for the benefit of Africa's inhabitants, which would resonate with the perennial proclamations of commitment. We propose that there were three brief moments. One such moment was in 1995–6 when the OAU, through the agency of the national governments of South Africa and Nigeria, revealed a disposition to present a pan-African agenda on HIV/

AIDS. The second moment was in the years 2000–2 when the OAU formulated a collective position that included demands for international support alongside collaborative endeavours, backed by the advocacy for action contained in the 2001 Abuja declaration. The third moment was in 2006 when the second special summit in Abuja provided a detailed position to enable universal access of Africans to HIV and tuberculosis treatment and sexual and reproductive health services. This is a sorry record: nineteen years of declarations and four to five years of action.

So what has the AU contributed to the effort of international agencies, national governments, NGOs and civil society in Africa? There is little to suggest that the AU has substantiated its professed leadership and commitment. Instead, the AU reflects all that is wrong with executive leadership in Africa since the early 1980s. The OAU's 1992 declaration asserted the claims to leadership of the collected heads of state. There was no ambivalence in the phrasing. Commitment was clearly defined (for example, 'giving our fullest political commitment'; 'using our leadership position'; 'make AIDS a top priority'). There were bold assertions (for example, 'By the end of 1992, each one of us will be publicly recognised as the leader of the fight against AIDS in one's own country'). There were definitive goals to be achieved during the following two years (for example, total ['100%'] education on HIV; national AIDS plans; co-ordination of action plans with research; allocation of necessary funding). All these claims were substantiated with the specification of responsibility and agency in the use of the term 'we' and, in one clause, 'all of us'. Similarly emphatic intentions and sentiments have been expressed regularly thereafter, particularly in 2001 and 2006. This has an appearance of transformational leadership, yet in reality it is bereft of substance and merely repeated with no reflection on effect.

In other words, the AU's declarations and decisions belie the impression of collective, laudable leadership by Africa's heads of state. First, it is not hard to see that the impression is sustained by the efforts of two heads of state, Olusegun Obasanjo and Abdoulaye Wade of Senegal. Their interventions lie behind the occasional developments in the AU's deliberations on HIV/AIDS. Furthermore, their interventions reveal a systemic agenda as well an agenda established by their predecessors. In short, they displayed transformational leadership.[24] Second, there are evident lapses after each intervention, as expressed in the lack of substantive development in the AU's deliberations on HIV/AIDS until the next inspirational events (for example, the United Nations assembly in 2001 and the Abuja summits). The lapse in the last three years is particularly telling. We refer here to the world now being in an era of HIV/AIDS management, as opposed to reacting to a little-understood health catastrophe, and in a context of ever-changing criteria to assess progress as opposed to one of stating and reiterating what should and needs to be done. Third, the AU's endorsement of internal advocacy by a group of peers (via AIDS Watch Africa) contradicts the stated commitments and decisions of the heads of state. It is on this basis that we contend that the AU has practised incidental leadership, as summarised in our judgement of 'nineteen years of declarations and four to five years of action'.

In metaphorical terms, Africa's 'heads' of state talk frequently about common symptoms of illness in their respective 'bodies' and how they need to mobilise the bodies' resources to deal with the illness. However, they have not mobilised the resources as they said they would. The exception was when these 'heads' have called upon the 'heads' of other states (donor governments and international health agencies) to provide assistance with the resources they have mobilised from their own 'bodies'.

The disjunction between the leadership proclaimed by Africa's heads of state via the AU and what has been practised reverberates down throughout regional and national political structures. There are regional government agencies – for example the Southern African Development Community (SADC) and the East African Community (EAC) – which, like the AU, are designed to foster co-operation. However, also like the AU, they can show little beyond producing documents to the effect of saying what national governments should do to curtail the HIV pandemic. This is in stark contrast to the substantive efforts of international agencies and national and regional

NGOs in Africa to assist these regional agencies in their work. For instance, international donor agencies have regional programmes which, in southern Africa, provide direct support to SADC and which encourage NGOs to work with SADC. At national levels of government, the disjunction is visible in the gaps between principles and practice of government policies. Most countries now endorse political democracy and a human rights agenda which, in the field of healthcare, are aligned to the principles of the WHO model of decentralised health services and refinements over time (for example, co-ordination and integration of services and a people-centred approach) (WHO 2006a, 2006b, 2006c). These principles are often reflected in national legislation and in ratifications of United Nations conventions. However, there is a very patchy record of understanding within governments of what they have committed themselves to, let alone applications of the principles, policies and legislation (see, for example, Gerntholtz, Grant and Hanass-Hancock 2010). This is an underlying theme in various chapters in this book.

To illustrate further, Zambia used to have an independent entity within the central ministries, the Central Board of Health, to co-ordinate funding and programming. This was appropriate in terms of having national structures capable of co-ordinating government activities and overriding ministerial competition. It was closed in 2006, however, enabling the Ministry of Health to reassert its central status in the national response to HIV/AIDS.[25] In South Africa, the government emphasises partnerships with NGOs to broaden people's access to welfare services and to expand its home-based care programmes but these 'partnerships' amount to little more than funding support. There is little evidence of sound mechanisms to monitor and regulate the plethora of NGOs that have been established in the wake of government funding (Campbell et al. 2007; GTZ n.d.; Health Promotion Unit 2008; Potter 2010).

To be clear, our point here is that the patchy record is indefensible twenty-plus years after African acknowledgement of the threat posed by HIV/AIDS, in the context of African governments' frequent proclamations of a collective leadership role and their regular endorsement of sound means to contain the pandemic and, as importantly, in view of the vast financial and technical support provided by international agencies and the initiatives of civil society organisations. Collectively, African governments have shown a lack of accountability to the continent's inhabitants. Claims of leadership and interest in citizens' welfare count for little in the relative absence of decisive action to apply new knowledge and to adapt to changing terms for debates and decision-making on strategy and policy. Elaboration of the ideologies of political democracy and human rights in Africa encourages critical assessment of governments in terms of whether they are doing 'right' or wrong' in dealing with the HIV/AIDS pandemic. These ideologies presume a relationship of trust and mutual dependency between citizen and government. However, the collective record of African governments reveals failure to substantiate their professed concern and interest in the health of their citizens and, hence, disregard for their welfare.

The net result is denial of citizenship. The effects are experienced in daily life, as we noted earlier, as people face real difficulties in gaining access to healthcare in their own and other African countries. The real effects of this denial lead us to take the point further. Borrowing from Derrida (1997), we contend that the citizen is an 'enemy' in the eyes of African governments. Again, to be clear, we are not saying that governments consciously regard citizens as their enemies. We find Derrida's work useful in this instance because it is helpful in understanding the travesty of the multitude of AIDS-related deaths in Africa. That these deaths have occurred and are allowed to continue is, in Derrida's terms, negation of the enemy (1997: 112–37). The death of many people gets rid of witnesses to governments' responsibility to citizens' right to life. Equally, governments can mitigate public outrage via rhetoric, such as that espoused by the AU, backed by reference to their endorsement of appropriate policies and mechanisms to contain the pandemic. Occasional admissions of guilt, such as acknowledging a slow response, offset by claims about constraints such as lack of resources, further negate public concern.

It is, objectively, a contradictory stance and the façade is wearing very thin. This leads us to consider why it has been sustained for so long. Here, we recognise that such hypocrisy cannot be the preserve of governments alone. The denial of citizenship has also been endorsed in societal prejudices about those infected with HIV. For instance, it is evident in presumptions of homosexuality as a cause of infection, the effect being to portray the person as 'abnormal' in relation to heterosexual norms. Likewise it is evident in many religious (particularly Christian) portrayals of infected, heterosexual persons as 'sinners'. In this book, Chapters 5 and 8 draw attention to these prejudices. Objective description of this rhetoric in terms of 'stigma' and 'discrimination' obscures the denial of humanity in daily life. Furthermore, such prejudice is in accord with popular portrayal of society at war with HIV/AIDS. Once infection with the virus was seen to lead inevitably to death and to be occurring across the world, it was a short jump to perceive a major threat to human existence, thence to the need for a concerted response and so, to martial terms such as 'combating HIV'. The problem with the war terminology is the potential confusion over whether society is fighting an external enemy or itself; indeed, whether the fight is against the virus or its hosts.

We have qualified our critique of African governments' collective rhetoric on HIV/AIDS because one can only begin to make sense of what has happened and is happening by acknowledging the ever-changing conditions for critical assessment. We outlined these considerations earlier in terms of how criticism of African governments is exacerbated or dispelled not only by past records but also, whether they show continuity and consistency (governments can and do 'lose the plot'), how they respond to foreseeable demands and whether they appreciate new criteria for assessing progress. This perspective brings into relief the dearth of sound executive leadership in Africa. There are few heads of state who have questioned explanations of HIV/AIDS that externalise the problem and who have taken to heart the imperative of collective responsibility and mutual support. This is the kernel of the critiques presented in the following chapters.

Notes

1. The following chapters show that this does not mean all interpretations and uses of the partial, yet ever-expanding knowledge are equally valid.

2. Perspectives on responses to HIV/AIDS are coloured now by the alacrity of government responses to threats such as SARS in 2003–4 and, more recently, swine flu.

3. We view such prejudice, as Lawson infers, to be a function of denial, which is one stage in psycho-social reactions to disease.

4. From a scientific perspective, sexual intercourse is a *means* of HIV transmission, not a *cause*. Causes are, from a medical viewpoint, the biological, biochemical and physical conditions that facilitate transmission of the virus during sexual intercourse. From a social science viewpoint, causes are the socio-economic and behavioural factors that increase the presence of pertinent biological, biochemical and physical conditions for transmission of the virus.

5. Postgraduate students in the Department of Anthropology at the University of Cape Town, where one of the authors was completing his Master's thesis at the time, were offered research funding (remarkably large sums in the minds of the students and staff) to conduct research on the 'new' disease. There was little interest, the students being convinced largely by discussion amongst themselves that the funding and focus were not appropriate in view of the marked lack of research funding for and inability of the health services to contain common, highly prevalent diseases such as tuberculosis and measles.

6. HIV incidence, the number of new infections over a given period of time, is another means but difficult to measure. HIV prevalence, incidence and mortality rates are derived from sophisticated models that provide estimates. The models are known to be inaccurate and, though regularly refined and recalibrated to improve the quality of information, the imprecision of the estimates is often cause for disputes (Whiteside 2008: 14–21).

7. Mr Mbeki stated that 'HIV does not cause AIDS'. His was the prominent voice of the government but he was supported by twelve of the thirteen ministers in the Cabinet; only one publicly contradicted him.

8. Prostitution was legalised in 1969. Controls, including registration of prostitutes, mandatory quarterly medical checks and general surveillance and treatment of sexually transmitted illnesses, have been governed by the Bureau of Venereal Disease since 1970 (Putzel 2003; Willems 2009).

9. Botswana is a well-known exception for reasons noted earlier. However, anecdotal reports in 2007 suggested that a lack of skilled administrators was constraining the public health system from achieving its potential.

10. This does not mean they were ineffective, only that results were and still are difficult to measure and possibly their contribution requires a long time frame to become evident.

11. Expectations also increase as new technological improvements become known; for instance, the introduction of highly active antiretroviral therapy and pill formulations that obviate the need for refrigeration – a critical factor for treatment in many rural areas of Africa.

12. It can be argued also that an increase in HIV prevalence in the short term (three to five years), rather than a decline, coupled with a decrease in AIDS mortality rates would signify an effective treatment programme. In the mid-term (approximately five to ten years) measures of a consistently effective programme would be an ongoing decrease in death rates, a marked drop in the number of new infections (incidence) and, towards the end of the period, a gradual levelling of prevalence (a slower rate of increase).

13. A Malawian official who gave the keynote speech at a function during a conference in Bloemfontein (in November 2007) underpinned his speech with the acronym 'KISS' (Keep it Simple Stupid). He used it to explain changes in his government's strategy in the light of reviews that had highlighted environmental challenges (for example, topography and distances) for implementing comprehensive prevention and treatment programmes and concerns about the reliance on external funding.

14. The Malawian government gained notoriety in the international media for the same reason in 2010.

15. Southern Sudan obtained independence in 2011 and has joined the AU, thereby increasing the number of member states to 54.

16. This method of analysis is known as periodisation in rhetoric research methodology. This first assumes the existential nature of declarations before we can consider them analysable or usable (Fowler 1972: 487–509; White 1980).

17. The formulation of the United Nations Millenium Development Goals influenced the tenor of the AU's decisions and declarations this decade (Adebajo, Adedeji and Landsberg 2007). Likewise, the same may be said of continental development plans arising from initiatives (acknowledged in OAU and AU deliberations) by South Africa's president at the time, Thabo Mbeki and Senegal's president, Abdoulaye Wade. We refer here to the New Partnership for Africa's Development (NEPAD), driven largely by Mbeki and the OMEGA Plan, prepared by Wade (Wade 2001; Gelb 2002).

18. This is due to the Abuja summit being a landmark in Africa during a period of intensive international advocacy to formulate concerted global commitment (expressed at the United Nations General Assembly in 2001). This advocacy included the launch of the International Partnership against AIDS in Africa in 2000, which produced an 'African Consensus and Plan of Action: Leadership to Overcome HIV/AIDS' (UNAIDS 2008: 105-6, 110, 118-20, 128-9).

19. AIDS Watch Africa was transferred to the AU in 2004 (AWA 2006).

20. For example, 'Foster and strengthen community, national, regional and continental leadership and strong political commitment that builds on and

strengthens existing African institutions at all levels, including civil society institutions'; 'Integrate the control of HIV/AIDS with broader efforts to combat poverty and food insecurity and fostering development, whilst recognizing the urgency and exceptionality of the HIV and AIDS response'; 'Put people at the centre of the HIV and AIDS response'; 'Adopt gender centred approaches'; 'Respect of human rights'; 'Ensure mutual accountability'; 'Maintain an unwavering commitment' (AU 2006a: 4).

21. The AU website (www.african-union.org) contains a detailed record of ordinary sessions and associated meetings.

22. 'Harmonization' is a common term used by the Joint United Nations Programme on HIV/AIDS (UNAIDS) and European donor agencies (although not agencies in the United States) in promoting co-ordination of their own and other agencies regional HIV/AIDS-oriented programmes.

23. AIDS Watch Africa is acknowledged in other assembly reports (see, for example, AU 2005, 2006c).

24. In the case of Obasanjo, the limitation is that his statesmanship on the continental stage is not reflected at home, in view of Nigeria's escalating HIV/AIDS epidemic.

25. In this case, it is arguable whether the change in structures improved Zambia's capacity to curtail the national HIV/AIDS epidemic. For instance, it could be said that the country's expansion of its ARV programme occurred in spite of that change and because of the large-scale funding obtained in 2004–5 and in 2008–9 from the American government and The Global Fund to Fight AIDS, Tuberculosis and Malaria (GFATM).

References

Adebajo, A., A. Adedeji and C. Landsberg (eds). 2007. *South Africa in Africa: The Post-Apartheid Era*. Pietermaritzburg: University of KwaZulu-Natal Press.

Anderson, B. 1998. *The Spectre of Nations: Nationalism, Southeast Asia and the World*. London: Verso.

Altman, D. 1986. *AIDS and the New Puritanism*. New York: Pluto Press.

AU (African Union). 2003. 'Decisions and Declarations'. Assembly of the African Union Second Ordinary Session, 10–12 July, Maputo, Mozambique. Addis Ababa: AU.

———. 2005. 'Decisions and Declarations'. Assembly of the African Union Fourth Ordinary Session, 30–31 January, Abuja, Nigeria. Addis Ababa: AU.

———. 2006a. 'Universal Access to HIV/AIDS, Tuberculosis and Malaria Services by 2010: Africa's Common Position to the UN General Assembly Special Session on AIDS' (June 2006). Report of Special Summit of the AU on HIV/AIDS, Tuberculosis and Malaria, Abuja, Nigeria. Addis Ababa: AU.

———. 2006b. 'Update on HIV/AIDS Control in Africa'. Report (Sp/EX.CL/ ATM/3 (I) for the Special Summit of the AU on HIV/AIDS, Tuberculosis and Malaria, 2–4 May, Abuja, Nigeria.

———. 2006c. 'Decisions, Declarations and Recommendation'. Assembly of the African Union Sixth Ordinary Session, 23–24 January, Khartoum, Sudan. Addis Ababa: AU.

———. 2006d. 'Decisions and Declarations'. Assembly of the African Union Seventh Ordinary Session, 1–2 July, Banjul, The Gambia. Addis Ababa: AU.

———. 2008. 'Decisions, Declarations, Tribute and Recommendation'. Assembly of the African Union Eleventh Ordinary Session, 30 June – 1 July, Sharm El-Sheikh, Egypt. Addis Ababa: AU.

———. 2010. 'Decisions'. Executive Council Seventeenth Ordinary Session, 19–23 July, Kampala, Uganda. Addis Ababa: AU.

AWA (AIDS Watch Africa). 2006. 'Minutes of AIDS Watch Africa (AWA)'. Addis Ababa: AU.

Bärngihausen, T., D.E. Bloom and S. Humair. 2007. 'Human Resources for Treating HIV/AIDS: Needs, Capacities and Gaps'. *AIDS Patient Care and STDs* 21(11): 799–812.

Beck, E.J., N. Mays, A.W. Whiteside and J.M. Zuniga (eds). 2006. *The HIV Pandemic: Local and Global Implications.* Oxford: Oxford University Press.

Billig, M. 1991. *Ideology and Opinion.* London: Sage.

———. 1996. *Arguing and Thinking: A Rhetorical Approach to Social Psychology.* Cambridge: Cambridge University Press.

Bolland, J. and J. Wilson. 1994. 'Three Faces of Integrative Coordination: A Model of Inter-organizational Relations in Community Based Health and Human Services'. *Health Services Research Journal* 3: 341–66.

Brink, A. 2000. *Debating AZT: Mbeki and the AIDS Drug Controversy.* Pietermaritzburg: Open Books.

Butler, A. 2005. 'South Africa's HIV/AIDS Policy, 1994–2004: How Can It Be Explained'. *Africa Affairs* 104(417): 591–614.

Campbell, C. 2003. *'Letting Them Die': Why HIV/AIDS Prevention Programmes Fail.* Oxford: James Currey.

Campbell, C., Y. Nair, S. Maimane and Z. Sibiya 2007. 'Supporting People with AIDS and Their Caregivers in Rural South Africa: Possibilities and Challenges'. *Health & Place*: 1–12.

Chen, L., T. Evans, S. Anand, J. Boufford, H. Brown and M. Chowdhury. 2004. 'Human Resources for Health: Overcoming the Crisis'. *Lancet* 364 (9 449): 1984–90.

Department of Health. 2005. 'National HIV and Syphilis Prevalence Survey South Africa 2005'. Pretoria: Department of Health.

Derrida, J. 1997. *Politics of Friendship*. London: Verso.

Dorrington, R., D. Bradshaw and D. Budlender. 2002. 'HIV/AIDS Profile in the Provinces of South Africa: Indicators for 2002'. Cape Town: Centre for Actuarial Research, University of Cape Town.

Fowler, A. 1972. 'Periodization and Interart Analogies'. *New Literary History* 3(3): 487–509.

Gelb, S. 2002. *The New Partnership for Africa's Development (NEPAD): A Brief Overview*. Braamfontein: The Edge Institute.

Gerntholtz, L., K. Grant and J. Hanass-Hancock. 2010. 'Disability Rights, HIV & AIDS in Eastern and Southern Africa: A Review of International, Regional and National Commitments on Disability Rights in the Context of HIV & AIDS in Eastern and Southern Africa'. Durban: Health Economics and HIV/AIDS Research Division (HEARD), University of KwaZulu-Natal. Available at www.heard.org.za.

Goldacre, B. 2009. 'The Doctor Will Sue You Now'. Available at www.badscience.net/files/The-Doctor-Will-Sue-You-Now.pdf.

Grundlingh, L. 2001. 'A Critical Historical Analysis of Government Responses to HIV/AIDS in South Africa as Reported in the Media, 1983–1994'. Unpublished paper. Johannesburg: Department of Historical Studies, University of Johannesburg.

GTZ (Deutsche Gesellschaft für Technische Zusammenarbeit). n.d. (c.2003). 'Findings: HBC Baseline Survey, 2002–2003, Summary Report, Mpumulanga Rural Development Programme'.

Guillespie, S. (ed.). 2006. *AIDS, Poverty and Hunger: Challenges and Responses*. Washington, DC: International Food Policy Research Institute.

Hanefeld, J. and M. Musheke. 2009. 'What Impact Do Global Health Initiatives Have on Human Resources for Antiretroviral Treatment Roll-Out? A Qualitative Policy Analysis of Implementation Processes in Zambia'. *Human Resources for Health* 7: 8.

Hankin, C., K. Stanecki, P. Ghys and H. Marais. 2006. 'The Evolving HIV Pandemic'. In E.J. Beck, A. Mays, A.W. Whiteside and J.M. Zuniga (eds). *The HIV Pandemic: Local and Global Implications*. New York: Oxford University Press: 21–35.

Health Promotion Unit. 2008. 'Community-Based Care and Support for People Infected and Affected by HIV/AIDS in Region 8, Johannesburg' (abbreviated report). Johannesburg: Division of Public Oral Health and Health Promotion Unit, Schools of Public Health and Oral Health Sciences, University of the Witwatersrand.

HEARD (Health Economics and HIV/AIDS Research Division). 2009. 'Human Resources for Health in South Africa'. Available at www.heard.org.za.

HSRC (Human Sciences Research Council). 2009. 'South African National HIV Prevalence, Incidence, Behaviour and Communication Survey, 2008: A Turning Tide among Teenagers?' Cape Town: HSRC.

Huicho, L., R.W. Scherpbier, A.M. Nkowane and C.G. Victoria. 2008. 'How Much Does Quality of Child Care Vary between Health Workers with Differing Durations of Training? An Observational Multicountry Study'. *Lancet* 372: 910-6.

Illiffe, J. 2006. *A History of the African AIDS Epidemic*. Oxford: James Currey.

Lawson, L. 2008. *Side Effects: The Story of AIDS in South Africa*. Cape Town: Double Storey.

Lush, L., E. Darkoh and S.L. Ramotlhwa. 2006. 'Botswana'. In E.J. Beck, N. Mays, A.W. Whiteside and J.M. Zuniga (eds). *The HIV Pandemic: Local and Global Implications*. New York: Oxford University Press: 181-214.

Mangcu, X. 2008. *To the Brink: The State of Democracy in South Africa*. Pietermaritzburg: University of KwaZulu-Natal Press.

Meda, N., I. Ndoye, S. M'Boup, A. Wade, S. Ndiaye, C. Niang, F. Sarr, I. Diop and M. Careal. 1999. 'Low and Stable HIV Infection Rates in Senegal: Natural Course of the Epidemic or Evidence for Success of Prevention'. *AIDS* 13: 1397-405.

Mills, A., J. Vaughan, D. Smith and I. Tabibzadeh (eds). 1990. *Health System Decentralization: Concepts, Issues and Country Experience*. Geneva: World Health Organization.

OAU (Organisation of African Unity). 1991. 'Declarations and Resolutions Adopted by the Twenty-Seventh Ordinary Session of the Assembly of Heads of State and Government, 3-5 June, Abuja, Nigeria'. OAU Secretariat.

———. 1992. 'Declarations and Resolutions Adopted by the Twenty-Eighth Ordinary Session of the Assembly of Heads of State and Government, 28-30 June 1993, Dakar, Senegal'. OAU Secretariat.

———. 1994. 'Declarations and Resolutions Adopted by the Thirtieth Ordinary Session of the Assembly of Heads of State and Government, 13-15 June, Tunis, Tunisia'. OAU Secretariat.

———. 1995. 'Declarations and Resolutions Adopted by the Thirty-First Ordinary Session of the Assembly of Heads of State and Government, 26-28 June, Addis Ababa, Ethiopa'. OAU Secretariat.

———. 1996. 'Declarations, Resolutions and Decisions Adopted by the Thirty-Second Ordinary Session of the Assembly of Heads of State and Government, 8-10 July, Yaoundé, Cameroon'. OAU Secretariat.

———. 1997. 'Declarations and Decisions Adopted by the Thirty-Third Ordinary Session of the Assembly of Heads of State and Government, Harare, Zimbabwe'. OAU Secretariat.

———. 1998. 'Declarations and Decisions Adopted by the Thirty-Fourth Ordinary Session of the Assembly of Heads of State and Government, 8-10 June, Ouagadougo, Burkina Faso'. OAU Secretariat.

———. 2000. 'Declarations and Decisions Adopted by the Thirty-Sixth Ordinary Session of the Assembly of Heads of State and Government, 10-12 July, Lome, Togo'. OAU Secretariat.

————. 2001a. 'Abuja Declaration on HIV/AIDS, Tuberculosis and Other Related Infectious Diseases'. Available at www.un.org/ga/aids/pdf/abuja_declaration.pdf.

————. 2001b. 'Decisions and Declarations Adopted by the Thirty-Seventh Ordinary Session/Fifth Ordinary session of the AEC (African Economic Community), 9-11 July, Lusaka, Zambia'. OAU Secretariat.

Ogundiran, A., B. Fatumbi and B.T. Costantinos. 2006. 'Nigeria'. In E.J. Beck, N. Mays, A.W. Whiteside and J.M. Zuniga (eds). *The HIV Pandemic: Local and Global Implications*. New York: Oxford University Press: 215-27.

Pisani, E. 2008. *The Wisdom of Whores: Bureaucrats, Brothels and the Business of AIDS*. London: Granta.

Poku, N. and A. Whiteside. 2004. 'Global Health and the Politics of Governance: An Introduction'. In N. Poku and A. Whiteside (eds). *Global Health and Governance: HIV/AIDS*. London: Palgrave Macmillan: 1-5.

Potter, L. 2010. 'Newcastle Social Marketing Project: Phase 2 of the Amajuba Child Health & Well-Being Research Project (ACHWRP)', HEARD Research Report. Health Economics and HIV/AIDS Research Division (HEARD), University of KwaZulu-Natal, Durban.

Preda, A. 2005. *AIDS, Rhetoric and Medical Knowledge*. Cambridge: Cambridge University Press.

Putzel, J. 2003. 'Institutionalising an Emergency Response: HIV/AIDS and Governance in Uganda and Senegal', report submitted to the Department for Institutional Development.

Quinlan, T. and S. Willan. 2004. 'Finding Ways to Contain the HIV/AIDS Epidemic: South Africa 2004-5'. In J. Daniel and R. Southall (eds). *State of the Nation Review 2004*. Pretoria: HSRC.

Schneider, H. 1998. 'The Politics behind AIDS: The Case of South Africa', presentation to the Twelfth World AIDS Conference, Geneva.

Siedel, G. and L. Vidal. 1997. 'The Implications of "Medical", "Gender in Development" and Culturalist Discourses for HIV/AIDS Policy in Africa'. In C. Shore and S. Wright (eds). *Anthropology of Policy: Critical Perspectives on Governance and Power*. London: Routledge: 59-87.

Simms, C., P.S. Sow and E. Sy. 2006. 'Senegal'. In E.J. Beck, N. Mays, A.W. Whiteside and J.M. Zuniga (eds). *The HIV Pandemic: Local and Global Implications*. New York: Oxford University Press: 228-39.

Stein, Z. and A. Zwi. 1990. *Action on AIDS in Southern Africa: Proceedings of Maputo Conference on Health in Transition in Southern Africa, April 9-16*. New York: Committee for Health in Southern Africa (CHISA), HIV Centre for Clinical and Behavioural Studies, New York State Psychiatric Institute and Columbia University.

UN (United Nations). 2004. 'A More Secure World: Our Shared Responsibility: Report on High-Level Panel on Threats, Challenges and Change'. New York: UN.

UNAIDS (Joint United Nations Programme on HIV/AIDS). 2004. 'Three Ones Principles: Coordination of National Responses to HIV AIDS Guiding Principles for National Authorities and their Partners'. Geneva: UNAIDS.

———. 2005. 'The Three Ones in Action: Where We Are and Where We Go from Here'. Geneva: UNAIDS.

———. 2008. 'UNAIDS: The First 10 Years'. Geneva: UNAIDS.

Wade, A. 2001. 'OMEGA Plan for Africa'. Available at www.sarpn.org/NEPAD/Omega.pdf.

Walt, G., J. Shiffman, H. Schneider, M. Susan, B. Ruairí and L. Gilson. 2008. 'Doing Health Policy Analysis: Methodological and Conceptual Reflections and Challenges'. *Health Policy and Planning* 2(6): 58–67.

Weinel, M. 2005. 'AIDS Policy in South Africa: Between Denial and Action', working paper, German Overseas institute.

White, E. 1980. 'Rhetoric as Historical Configuration'. In E. White (ed.). *Rhetoric in Transition: Studies in the Nature and Uses of Rhetoric*. University Park: Pennsylvania State University Press: 7–20.

Whiteside, A. 2008. *HIV/AIDS: A Very Short Introduction*. Oxford: Oxford University Press.

Whiteside, A.A. Whalley and S. Naysmith. 2007. 'Reviewing "Emergencies" for Swaziland: Shifting the Paradigm to a New Era'. National Emergency Response Council on HIV/AIDS, Mbabane and Health Economics and HIV/AIDS Research Division (HEARD), University of KwaZulu-Natal, Durban.

WHO (World Health Organization). 2003. 'World Health Report (Shaping the Future)'. Geneva: WHO.

———. 2006a. 'The Global Shortage of Health Workers and its Impact'. Available at www.who.int/mediacentre/factsheets/fs302/en/index.html.

———. 2006b. *The World Health Report 2006: Working together for health*. Geneva: World Health Organisation.

———. 2006c. 'Taking Stock: Health Worker Shortages and the Response to AIDS'. Available at www.who.int/hiv/pub/advocacy/ttr/en/index.html.

———. 2008. 'World Health Report: Primary Health Care – Now More Than Ever'. Geneva: WHO.

Willan, S. 2004. 'Briefing: Recent Changes in the South African Government's HIV/AIDS Policy and its Implementation'. *African Affairs* 103: 109–17.

Willems, S. 2009. 'The Importance of Interdisciplinary Collaborative Research in Responding to HIV/AIDS Vulnerability in Rural Senegal'. *African Journal of AIDS Research* 8(4): 433–42.

Wilson, K., J. Cohen-Kohler and A. Whiteside. 2008. 'The "Price is Right"? Promoting Local Production for ARVs in Sub-Saharan Africa'. *EuroHealth* 14(2): 29–32.

2

What Type of Leadership is Required to Combat Complex Global Challenges such as the HIV and AIDS Pandemic?

Judith Flick

This chapter explores what type of leadership it takes to contain the HIV pandemic at country, organisational and individual levels of intervention. The implicit argument is that collective leadership is possible and needs to happen across sectors to be effective. The working definition of leadership is that 'at its core, leadership is about shaping and shifting how individuals and groups attend to and subsequently respond to a situation' (Scharmer 2007). In other words, one of the key functions of leadership is to hold the space in which the problems and aspirations (of individuals, society and organisations) are respectively understood systemically and achieved. Part of the leadership responsibility is to bring together individuals and communities around these issues and help them to find appropriate answers for their diverse needs. The first step is that leaders themselves carry the issues at heart. A detailed description of the process is provided and illustrated through an example from Zambia.

The challenge
The first question that arises when looking at leadership in relation to HIV and AIDS in southern Africa is: why did it take so long for gifted,

committed leaders and liberation fighters such as Thabo Mbeki and Nelson Mandela to recognise the threat that the HIV pandemic constituted to the continued existence of the people who elected them into power? What held them back from taking prompt and appropriate action when they held positions of power that had the potential for making positive changes?

Second, millions of dollars have been spent on HIV and AIDS by multinationals, local and international non-governmental organisations (NGOs) and foundations (such as the Bill and Melinda Gates Foundation), Susan Thompson and Warren Buffett, and (ex-) presidents such as Bill Clinton. There was a six-fold increase in donations to low- and middle-income countries from 2001–7 and yet we do not see effects in terms of an overall reduction in the numbers of infections, deaths and related suffering of the people infected and affected by HIV and AIDS (UNAIDS 2008). What would it take to turn this around?

Third, how can we learn from the numerous examples of personal and organisational selfless, ingenious and locally appropriate responses? How can we deal with the tension between the spread and scale of the pandemic on the one hand and, on the other, the need for diverse and locally sustained responses?

These were the three questions that set off my search for inclusive, diverse, efficient and sustainable answers to the HIV pandemic. This was in 2003 when I was serving as Oxfam Great Britain's regional director for southern Africa. My aspiration to address these questions led to the establishment of a Global Centre of Learning on HIV and AIDS and Oxfam Great Britain asked me to become the Global Lead on HIV and AIDS. I served in this role from 2004–7, in addition to being regional director for southern Africa.

What struck me when I returned to Africa after living and working in Latin America for seven years was that the debate and response to the HIV pandemic had not changed significantly in that time. In spite of the significant drop in the price of antiretroviral drugs,[1] the drugs had not been made available to those who needed them most; less than 50% of young people had comprehensive knowledge about HIV and its prevention and even those who were aware resisted the thought of knowing their status or changing their behaviours accordingly (UNAIDS 2008).

I thought that my ignorance about the lack of progress was circumstantial: one can live in Latin America under the illusion that the battle is won and that life goes on as before. In Africa, I realised soon enough that nothing was further from the truth and that a different type of response was needed. What were we missing? I was aware of the overall funding gap. For example, the gap in funds to provide enough condoms across sub-Saharan Africa was at least US$2 billion (Hunter 2004: 32). However, the bigger problem was probably that funds did not reach the places where they were most needed. While private donations from Buffet, Clinton, Bush and Gates were dominating the global media, local NGOs were struggling to get money for very valuable and honourable work. Communities were left to look after people suffering with HIV on a voluntary basis and condoms were nowhere to be found in the villages I visited in Malawi, Zambia, Angola or Mozambique. People were using used sugar bags to wash their dead in the absence of surgical gloves that cost ten US cents a pair. Despite the establishment of institutions such as The Global Fund to Fight AIDS, Tuberculosis and Malaria (GFATM), officials at national and district levels in the countries I was visiting did not know about their existence. In cases where a few were aware of the existence of such institutions, people did not seem to have the capacity to write and submit credible proposals to obtain the needed funds. Global campaign organisations such as Oxfam Great Britain had difficulties arguing for more donations or, at least, for receipt of funds already pledged by international institutions and countries. The general sentiment was that countries and organisations eligible for the donations did not demonstrate the capacity to use existing money efficiently and effectively.

I was told that the funding channels were blocked: funding was available globally, but did not reach the local organisations responsible for the implementation of programmes. Meanwhile poverty was on the increase and dancing a deadly tango with the disease. This was not a new problem: a significant part of the NGO sector is always trying to address the lack of institutional capacity of local organisations. And yet, only some of this work seemed effective. In turn, NGOs were pointing in the direction of (local) governments. The capacity of the public health system was completely overburdened or simply absent and the political will of the government was the ultimate stumbling block.

Still others were arguing that the main obstacle was socio-cultural: after all these years of confrontation with the disease, people were still in a state of denial, including some prominent political leaders such as Thabo Mbeki. In his address to the International AIDS Conference (2000), for example, Mbeki reiterated his view that HIV was not wholly responsible for AIDS, leading hundreds of delegates to walk out on his speech. On another occasion, he turned the debate into a racial issue:

> 'I will not keep quiet while others whose minds have been corrupted by the disease of racism accuse us, the black people of South Africa, Africa and the world, as being, by virtue of our Africanness and skin colour, lazy, liars, foul-smelling, diseased, corrupt, violent, amoral, sexually depraved, animal-istic, savage and rapist' . . . Mr Mbeki's language disconcerted some of his own supporters, as he continued with the accusation that certain whites regarded blacks as 'rampant sexual beasts, unable to control our urges, unable to keep our legs crossed, unable to keep it in our pants' (*Sydney Morning Herald* 2004).

This was a disturbing response from a leader. The nationalist spirit and rebuttal of stereotypes of Africa and Africans, especially from the North, still preclude some leaders from appreciating the solutions that are readily available to them. Many people on the ground seem to be able to think creatively and go out of their way to make a difference. For example, I know a senior Catholic priest (name withheld) who often exhorted his congregation during counselling sessions about the use of condoms in their marital sexual relationships saying: 'Do not sin, but if you must, sin with a conscience' and:

> Don't have extramarital relationships and use your sexual drive
> for the procreation of children, but if you can't avoid having
> extramarital sex, then use a condom. What's more, if you have
> contracted HIV through extra marital relationships, take
> responsibility for your wife's life and the future of your children
> by using a condom when having sex with her.

Not that the priest would under normal circumstances condone sin, but through this approach, he was able to balance two important Catholic principles, protection of life and faithfulness in marriage, in a way that resonated with the present reality. When asked how this shift had happened he explained that it was informed by his practice. For a long time he had felt that the dogmatic position of the church was not responding to the needs of its (faithful) followers. This disconnection had made him feel unable to do his job. He and some colleagues had subsequently started to question the appropriateness of their leaders' responses under these particular circumstances. They had gathered and decided to approach the situation differently; in essence, with respect to the fundamental beliefs of their church but also with a pragmatic outlook on life.

Stigma and denial can fall away and leadership is triggered when people dare to open themselves to the reality they face, to align their organisational responses with it and, subsequently, to translate this knowledge into action in their personal lives, communities, institutions and beyond. It seemed to me that this was needed in all ambits of life: the private, public and civic sector and, more so, in a combined effort of these sectors. Pointing in the direction of one actor, whether private, public or civic, would not work as a solution. Collaboration would be needed. This was informed by the realisation that the underlying causes of the disease were intertwined and jointly responsible for the way the pandemic was spreading. Isolating one factor, whether economic, political, socio-cultural or infrastructural, would not do justice to the underlying system and a systemic approach was needed (Senge 1999). Finally, it was also increasingly clear that this pandemic – although not new any longer – was the first of its kind.

Although repeated waves of many other diseases – plague, influenza, tuberculosis, cholera, syphilis – have swept the world since the turn of the twentieth century, HIV/AIDS is the first epidemic of **a totally new disease** since the 1400s. It is the first global pandemic to begin after medicine crossed the threshold to modernity in the 1950s, gaining the laboratory capacity to identify a disease and its cases quickly, the field capacity to prevent its spread, the data systems needed to track epidemic growth virtually as it occurs (Hunter 2004: 21).

Hence, I felt that the array of present solutions would only address the effects of the disease. It would not bring about a breakthrough in the underlying system that could shift some of the more fundamental causes. For that to happen a new type of approach was needed, led by people who dared to look reality in the eye, dared to challenge the status quo, including present forms of collaboration across sectors, out of a sense of collective responsibility.

Defining the leadership gap
A key question then becomes: How can we create environments where these types of responses can emerge? My search brought me to ask: What brings about the kind of leadership that opens its eyes to what is at stake, without fear of repercussions from the status quo and is also capable of shifting the attention of others towards what is evident? Leadership is service to communities on issues that matter most and lies at the heart of the pandemic, while collective leadership goes beyond rhetoric and drives meaningful action with an open mind and with respect for diversity.

The primary question has several facets to it. First, how do leaders get to focus on what truly matters to the people entrusted to them? What does it take to refocus attention in a constantly changing environment and not get stuck in dogmas of the past? Nelson Mandela, for example, did not choose HIV and AIDS as a main issue while in office. He only did so in 2006 after the death of his son (Blair 2005).

Second, what combination of leaders and leadership is required? Is it sufficient to have only high-level political leaders driving actions or, as is the case in Uganda (Kirungi 2001), should there be encouragement of leadership at all levels and sectors of society? Is there a place for personal leadership in all of this? What is the highest point of leverage?

Third, how do we find locally appropriate responses that respect the diversity of human needs and that build on the diversity of available resources from all sectors? And how do we deal with the tension between the speed and scale needed to combat HIV and AIDS globally on the one hand and, on the other, the complexity of human transformation processes and respect for diversity?

An example of an innovative approach to leadership in Zambia
In 2006 an initiative was underway in Zambia that was trying to address these questions through an innovative approach. It would lead to new inroads in addressing the role of media, ideas about opening up the debates about voluntary counselling and testing (VCT) and to new ways of using the leadership roles of former heads of state.

The goal of the initiative was to achieve a breakthrough in thinking and action regarding the HIV pandemic by applying a change strategy called 'The U-Process' (Scharmer 2007) and to explore whether the methodology was scalable and/or could be applied to other areas and regions. This implied:
- Applying innovative cross-institutional, cross-sectoral forms of collaboration in dealing with HIV;
- Using 'best practice' in the field of social development, such as local partnerships that create locally appropriate ways of sustaining and continuously adapting the initiative to the changing reality;
- Applying social 'technologies' such as 'deep listening', 'sensing', 'generative dialogue', 'connecting to Self', to understand the blockages from different perspectives (not only cognitively) and enabling participants to connect with the system that they were part of and to find a breakthrough;

- Devising prototype ways to address key blockages at individual, community, national and possibly global levels (Scharmer 2007).[2]

The initiative evolved through along five discernable stages: co-initiating, co-sensing, co-presencing, co-creating and co-evolving. Figure 2.1 below summarises the process and logic.

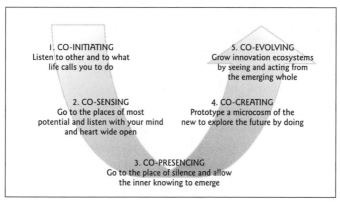

Figure 2.1   The U-change process (Scharmer 2007: 378).

During the first stage – co-initiation – which took place in July 2006, the geographical scope of the initiative, the initial purpose and intent, and the participants were identified. Invitations were extended to about twenty leaders who operated at national level and who had a strong commitment to controlling HIV and AIDS in Zambia. They had different backgrounds and experiences – in the business arena (microenterprises, mining); the arts and sports (fine art, football); NGOs (the Organization of People Living with HIV and AIDS, women's associations, trade unions, faith-based organisations); the government (National AIDS Council [NAC]); 'traditional' leadership (local chiefs) and the medical/education sector (a medical practitioner and a professor). Most of them had a track record in the field of HIV and

AIDS, and had arrived at the conclusion that 'more of the same solutions would not get Zambia on top of the disease'. They had heard of each other but seldom met. They had never worked together as a team.

Together they represented the stakeholders of the HIV and AIDS system. During their first meeting, they defined their vision:

- Happy Children: Children attend school. When they come home, there is someone who takes care of them. They have food and shelter and are looked after;
- Demystification of HIV/AIDS: An 'open society' where HIV/AIDS is seen as any other disease (and can therefore be talked about openly); where people infected with HIV do not have to face stigma and discrimination;
- Inspirational and servant leaders at all levels (not only at the top but in all sectors and among all people);
- Livelihoods: Fair Trade with countries outside Zambia and better distribution of livelihood within Zambia's own borders (Kalungu-Banda, Flick and Scharmer 2007: 10).

The participants arrived at this vision by looking into the present situation using creative visualisation techniques and by playing out scenarios of a desired future. There were, of course, referents to problems that the group perceived to be keeping the pandemic alive; notably, a failing social service system; stigma and discrimination; blind or unaccountable leadership; and insufficient livelihoods amongst a large part of the national population.

Subsequently this group decided to own the process to fulfil their vision. This decision occurred partly through self-organised meetings and partly through facilitated guidance. They established the Trust for Collective Action Against HIV and AIDS in Zambia (TCHAZa), asserting that their biggest asset was their collective commitment to embarking on a journey. They all understood that their strength lay in their collective wisdom and action, however remarkable their individual contributions were or had been previously.

The second stage, which took place between March and August 2007, consisted of a focused inquiry into the four components of their vision to prepare the ground for the creation of 'life examples', or prototypes for action. The group identified five areas where blockages to effective action could be or had been dispelled. Two principal criteria in this identification process were 'extreme users' of the system and 'places of most potential' for change. For example, to understand blockages in the livelihoods and education of children without caregivers, the group talked with children living on streets and leaders of organisations that took care of them. Similarly, to understand problems with and the potential of VCT, there were conversations with the users and the providers of VCT and, in particular, on unusual practices and services. For example, there was a conversation with the managers of a farm (who were also medical practitioners and very committed to the fight against HIV and AIDS) who had demanded that their staff test for HIV before committing to providing support and guaranteeing their jobs, no matter what the outcome of the test.

The objective was to define and present a refined description of the prototype constructive actions and what they would entail. A common consideration for each idea was a definition of the network of people who would be involved, the organisation or setting where it should take place, the core people who could drive and implement the ideas and actions, and the funding options. Furthermore, the group identified people who could dedicate time to inquiring into these areas through research, networking and dialogue. These 'inquirers' were trained and subsequently conducted their inquiry and sensing.[3] Each inquirer worked closely with his or her point person from the Trust (the leadership group). Every other week the whole group of inquirers and point persons from the Trust met to share what they had learned and what themes and questions were emerging from the ongoing inquiry process.

The third stage consisted of a workshop of the inquirers, trustees and invited guests to share the findings, reflect on them and to crystallise the key findings from the inquiry process. Four prototype ideas were generated; for example, facilitating the appointment of a special adviser on HIV and AIDS to the – now late – president of Zambia, Dr Mwanawasa. Like other presidential advisers, the adviser for HIV and AIDS would have daily access to the president, would represent him at important decision-making forums and help the president to demonstrate the leadership required on HIV/AIDS. In addition, the adviser would receive direct inputs from the government, civil society and business sectors, which, through representatives, would serve in a second-tier advisory capacity. Through the adviser, TCAHZa would have direct contact with the chairperson of the Cabinet committee on HIV and AIDS, whose role would be to formulate and implement policy on behalf of the president. This approach to influence policy and practice, from a cross-sectoral perspective, was well under way under during the era of the late president. Unfortunately it did not come to fruition, most likely because it did not fit the prescribed ways of operating within the existing structures.

Other prototypes explored the role of the media, different approaches to encourage people to go for testing and the role of the Zambian society in addressing the growing amount of children living without care on the streets. Some effects of these efforts are described below.

Exploring the leadership role of former African heads of state and African institutions

One of the early realisations of TCAHZa members was that a new type of leadership, dubbed 'inspirational leadership', was needed at every single level of society. The picture below draws on this idea by depicting 'apathetic' leadership represented by the man who prefers to lie in bed, rather than acting on the numerous possibilities that exist.

As a way of learning what inspirational leadership would look like at both a regional and a global level, TCAHZa, in partnership with the AIDS Public Health Communication Project (AIDSCOM), hosted a workshop for former heads of state in southern Africa to help them discover how they could use their status and influence HIV/AIDS interventions. That event inspired these leaders and Anglican bishops to join hands to go through similar processes.

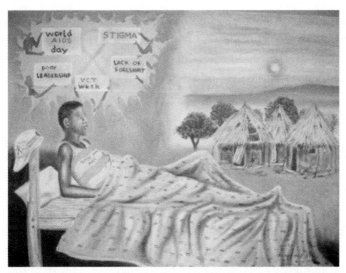

Picture by Gordon Shamulenge, a board member of the Trust
for Collective Action Against HIV and AIDS in Zambia.

Influencing the electronic and print media

In 2008, the Zambia National Broadcasting Corporation (ZNBC), the
country's leading TV and radio station, and public media increased
airtime dedicated to HIV and AIDS issues from less than 1% to 5%.
This was one of the highest percentages in Africa at the time. It was
made possible by the personal leadership of the chief executive of ZNBC,
Mr Jo Salasini, who was also a member of the African Broadcast Media
Partnership Against HIV (ABMPH) and a key member of TCAHZa.

Through their role in the Southern African Development
Community (SADC) Coalition of Broadcasting Corporations, the
ZNBC influenced other countries in SADC to follow suit. The project
saw a shift in the quality of reporting among key newspapers via the
methodologies transferred through the initiative to key people in the
print media houses. Initially, print media personnel thought that HIV
was no longer newsworthy, except in the event of information about a
cure. Many newspapers in Zambia began to find angles they never

imagined would be of interest to the readership; notably, human stories depicting positive attitudes, overcoming stigma, a shift in government policy and the sheer bravado of the people affected and infected frequently were headlines and on the front pages.

Building the local capacity of leaders and their institutions
The initiative led to the constitution of a group of twenty leaders across all sectors. Their biggest gain was a new type of consciousness and their biggest asset was a platform to connect them across traditional divides. Finding an adequate form and name for such an anomaly was a challenge. Zambian legislation recognised only two forms of NGOs: associations and trusts. Neither form was quite representative of the spirit of this group but they needed a way to comply with the regulatory framework for the establishment of their initiatives. The Trust succeeded in establishing a large platform for debate, networking and research. A number of cross-sectoral initiatives have emerged from a deeper understanding of the multidimensional nature of the pandemic.

The challenge for these leaders was to use their new skills and approaches in their own organisations. Several steps were taken to start this process, including the training of 25 people to be facilitators and focusing on senior management of organisations. Institutions that participated in the process included the ZNBC, Barclays Bank Zambia and the NAC.

How did this change come about?
The initiative was underpinned by Theory U, Leading from the Future as it Emerges (Scharmer 2007). It is a more elaborate explanation of a concept described a few years earlier by Senge et al. (2004). The focus of 'Theory U' is on the type of leadership required to find lasting solutions for complex global problems, such as climate change and HIV and AIDS. The theory is based on action research carried out over a period of ten years in the private, public and civic sectors. It built in teachings from the social liberation movements, wisdom traditions and theories about organisational learning and transformation across the globe.

Application of the theory directs participants in initiatives to develop seven capabilities for being members of multisectoral and multidisciplinary groups of leaders. Participants are taken together through a three-stage process, illustrated in Figure 2.2: 'Observe, observe, observe'; 'Retreat and reflect'; and 'Act in an instant'.

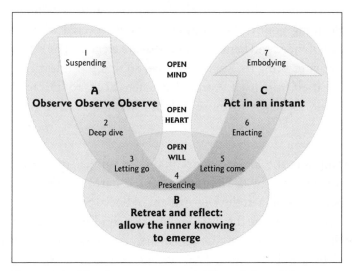

Figure 2.2   The three-stage process (adapted from Scharmer 2007: 45).

The first stage ('Observe, observe, observe'), is about taking in reality as it really is, not as we think it might be, hope it is or have been taught it should be. This requires 'suspending' judgement and mental models (step/capability 1) (Senge 1999) that prevent us from seeing without immediately attaching judgements to observations. It also requires a 'deep dive' (step/capability 2); that is, immersion in the reality being addressed. Good scientists practise this all the time; their education is geared towards observation based on data. But even for scientists this is not always easy because they have all been socialised into belief systems and use their judgement to make sense of everyday life. The premise is that truly innovative ways of changing a social system require seeing reality as it is and making connections. As Margaret Wheatley (2007: 93) put it:

> 'Information is what changes us' (Stafford Beer). When a system assigns meaning to data, when it 'in-forms' it, data then becomes information. To Create Better Health in a Living System, Connect it to More of Itself. When a system is failing, or performing poorly, the solution will be discovered within the system if more and better connections are created. The solution is always to bring the system together so that it can learn more about itself from itself. A troubled system needs to start talking to itself, especially to those it didn't know were even part of itself.

An example is the story of one of the 'inquirers' in the Zambian initiative, Evelyn Mwila-Mbulo. She was a part-time lecturer at the University of Zambia in the Department of Social Studies. Her starting point was to investigate the situation of street children, using traditional methods such as a questionnaire. At first, she would approach them guarded by a police officer. Her perception was that street children were aggressive drug abusers, difficult to approach and not to be trusted. However one day, when no police officer happened to be available to accompany her, she found herself having a conversation with an eight-year-old boy living on the streets. Her first surprise was his openness and vulnerability, not hers. Her second surprise was that he refused to be called 'street child'. Circumstances had driven him to the street. His perception was that he was not a 'street child' but a 'child living on the street'. Her third surprise came when he offered her a ten-Kwacha note and requested her to give it to her seven-year-old son to buy sweets for himself. At first, she refused to accept the money but he insisted. With this very simple but totally unexpected gesture of making a surprising connection with her (privileged) son, this eight-year-old boy turned her perceptions of 'street children' upside down. It gave a different meaning to the life of this boy, her son and how different economic strata in the Zambian society relate to each other.

Using Wheatley's phraseology, if 'seeing the system as it is and seeing the system from within' is to be part of a transformation process, the first stage has to mirror the system that wants to be established. This includes the establishment of new relationships, in a different way: a way that reflects the power relationships that can redirect the system in a different manner. The most effective way – maybe the only way – is if the key stakeholders of the system get a chance to see the system with fresh eyes, recognise their role in the present system and their transformative role by engaging with the system directly. They also need to learn to look 'through each others' eyes'; learn to see the interconnectedness of the different players, from different sectors, with different skills and experiences. Hence, if Evelyn had a chance to visit those children with other key players in the system, it could have led to a deeper and different connection between these players too. That is significant because unleashing a transformation requires more than one player, but not many; as Margaret Mead reportedly said: 'Never doubt that a small group of citizens can change the world. Indeed, it's the only thing that ever has' (Scharmer 2007).

'Seeing the system as it is' seems a simple act of engaging the citizenry, but the implications are vast. It implies that leaders cannot outsource the collection and analysis of data and information to others. They need such sources of information to determine where to look, what to look for and to ask the right questions. But they also need to engage more directly with the social system they are leading. How many leaders get a chance to do this? The further up the hierarchy they are, the more removed leaders are from the realities of life for the people they are leading. Sometimes this distance is cleverly orchestrated but often it is a simply due to the many demands placed on them. Ironically, it seems that their responsibilities are often what keeps them from being responsive to what really needs to be addressed.

When they have a chance to break through these shields it unleashes great potential for change. Scharmer's (2008) detailed analysis and description of profound change processes is instrumental in understanding the next steps of such a transformation process. He describes the need to 'let go' of familiar thinking (step 3), the need for reflection (step 4) and allowing something new to come to the fore (step 5).

To illustrate, Thabo Mbeki held on to his own views to interpret facts on HIV and AIDS; the Catholic priest mentioned earlier changed his way of thinking thereby allowing the emergence of a solution to his dilemma. Rather than revisiting his beliefs, Mbeki used facts about HIV and AIDS to reinforce his existing way of thinking. For example, his statement, 'accepting that HIV has hit our black population more than the whites, is like accepting that black men cannot control their natural drives and in a certain sense are still savages', was a reaffirmation of his views on the prevalence of racism. It was not an acknowledgement of the demographic patterns of the epidemic in South Africa nor even simply a questioning of the way demographic patterns were and continue to be presented in South Africa in public and scientific discourse (see Chapter 9 in this volume). Likewise, many religious people find comfort in thinking that HIV is a disease sent by God to punish those who have sinned. Facing the true nature of the pandemic is threatening precisely because it threatens existing beliefs and stimulates questioning of the structures and institutions built on those beliefs. In terms of the 'Theory U', this holding onto existing positions on issues and to the power derived from it (in terms of a sense of personal, emotional security and, more broadly, political authority) gets in the way of seeing what is required. What is required, in terms of the theory is 'presencing'.

The word 'presencing' is a blend of the two words 'presence' and 'sensing'. It refers to a state of being present and sensing the future that wants to emerge, connecting with one's purpose, letting go of the past and acting from one's highest future potential (Scharmer 2008: 468-9). Real transformation, whether at an individual level or collectively, whether in a small unit such as a family or a large company, will not last unless it is somehow connected with a deeper source of knowing. I know from my own experience how difficult it can be to detach oneself from the demands of a job, to stand back and reflect. Yet, when this is done, it reveals new insights that help move a situation forward much more effectively than simply ploughing through all the work piled on our desks. The same applies to 'letting come'. It requires trust in the process and in one's own capacity to crystallise what comes up.

We are more familiar with the sixth step – 'enacting', which is about representing a thought or concept visually. The trick is not to try to do this perfectly but simply to do it and use the 'draft' or first version as a basis to learn and refine it. The learning from the feedback on a simplified, even simplistic, first version is the main aim of this step. Feedback is generated through sharing with key stakeholders (amongst others the end-users) and applying it in real life. Subsequent versions lead to either a final product or to rejection of the whole idea if enacting shows that it is too simplistic or is more about existing beliefs than the reality of a situation.

Once there is a final version, one can turn to considering who or what organisation could use it, how, ways of marketing the idea and ways of funding the use. This step (step 7) is called 'embodiment'. This is a creative processes which construes complex global problems as requiring more than one agency to find suitable and sustainable solutions; hence, as in the Zambian case, the involvement from the start of a wide range of leaders and representatives of different sectors in society.

What is keeping leaders from taking these steps?
The U-process is not new to debates and knowledge on leadership. Most people are familiar with the process, what differs is the degree of conscious application among leaders. Those who recognise the steps know that it is a path to transform a situation, beliefs, institutions and themselves. A critical question, therefore, is: if this process is not invention but a discovery and, if it is effective to help understand and confront problems, then why do leaders not apply it more often? What are the obstacles that leaders face in applying this theory? Three things may get in their way at the left side of the 'U': the 'voice of judgement', the 'voice of cynicism' and the 'voice of fear' (Scharmer 2008).

The voice of judgement limits our ability to take in new information, because we see it in terms of what we have already learned to see. The voice of cynicism limits our ability to connect with our emotional intelligence because we sweep this aside with cynical comments or let others do that job for us. Finally, the voice of fear limits our ability to recognise the wisdom that surfaces out of fear of loss (money, power, worldly attachments). There are three further stumbling blocks as explained below:

> Moving down the left side of the U is about opening up and dealing with the resistance of thought, emotion, and will; moving up the right side is about intentionally reintegrating the intelligence of the head, the heart, and the hand in the context of practical applications. Just as the inner enemies on the way down the U represent the VOJ (voice of judgement), the VOC (voice of cynicism), and the VOF (voice of fear), the enemies on the way up the U are the three old methods of operating: executing without improvisation and mindfulness (reactive action); endless reflection without a will to act (analysis paralysis); and talking without a connection to source and action (blah-blah-blah). These three enemies share the same structural feature. Instead of balancing the intelligence of the head, heart, and hand, one of the three dominates – the will in mindless action, the head in endless reflection, the heart in endless networking (Scharmer 2008: 11).

So, if these pitfalls – the voices of judgement, cynicism and fear are so 'natural' and if our best practice in development is so hard to enact consistently and at scale, what are our chances of delivering on the leadership challenge? I don't have the answer but I do know, like others, what questions to ask and what steps to take.

Conclusion
The main question in this chapter is what kind of leadership it would take to turn the course of the HIV pandemic around in southern Africa. Three questions are central to this.

The first question is: How do leaders focus on issues that really matter to those that are entrusted to them? Or: How can leaders miss or ignore vital elements for the survival of their followers? The example used in this chapter suggests that a particular approach can be effective

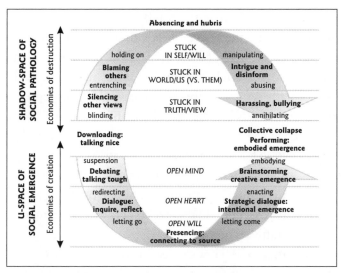

Figure 2.3   The U-space and the anti-space (Scharmer 2008: 282).

to create environments where leaders focus on what matters in a dynamic and constantly changing environment. Leaders demonstrate more responsive leadership when they are in a position that enables them to open up the mind, the heart and the will. This is facilitated by confrontational life experiences (for example, Kenneth Kaunda's son dying of AIDS) and/or carefully orchestrated sensing journeys (Scharmer 2008) whereby people can reconnect with the reality on the ground as it is evolving, without upfront judgement. It is important that sensing journeys are undertaken by the main players in the system, because the act of personal engagement is part of the process of transformation. Theory U not only provides a solid explanation for the multiple difficulties faced by leaders at all levels to successfully lead these types of social transformations, it also points to avenues that could be explored and developed more deliberately in order to create the type of leadership that is required to combat HIV and AIDS.

The second question is: What combination of leaders and leadership is required? Since HIV and AIDS is a complex multifaceted disease with underlying causes that cut across all sectors (economic, political, socio-cultural, infrastructural), any approach trying to shift the ground (not only the effects) needs to address the issue in a way that takes into account all of these angles. The constellation of leaders required to address such a complex issue needs to reflect the stakeholders of the system. In this case that would imply representatives from government, the NGO sector and the private sector. Organisations that want to be at the front of such transformation need to be able to create spaces where key stakeholders across all sectors can engage in a dialogue on an equal footing to generate new ideas. This requires suspension of judgement and cynicism about other sectors and the facilitation of spaces where these stakeholders can experiment without fear for loss of status or money.

The third question is: How can leaders respect the diversity of needs and values of societies in their response to the pandemic *and* deal with the scale of the pandemic at the same time? Bringing together such a diversity of players on an equal footing throughout the process will automatically lead to a more inclusive and diverse response. What remains to be answered is how scalable these approaches are. Responses that fit local needs and values have proven to be more effective and sustainable. The downside has always been that they are difficult to scale up.

The Zambian initiative did not go unnoticed in the Oxfam community. The organisation had to take risks, such as funding an open-ended process rather than a project with concrete deliverables, a process whereby all parties from all sectors were invited as equals around the table rather than around prescribed terms of reference defined upfront by one of the parties (usually the organisation who funds the initiative). This was against normal (good) practice. Innovation needs courage to be in the space that initially appears to be directionless or unproductive. Organisations want results and clear processes/ programmes. Innovation seems to emanate from spaces that are less defined and at times may seem wasteful. The people who were able to participate in the process or were able to look beyond the organisational mandate, usually reacted enthusiastically and some started replicating this process spontaneously in other areas. Those who did not participate or preferred to stick to rules and regulations were prone to reject the initiative and impose rigid standards. Asking people to suspend their judgement is one thing, asking an organisation to hold some rules and regulations loosely while waiting for the initiative to mature, is a different ball game.

The partners in the initiative faced the same challenges: they also took risks and had a hard time selling some of the intangible results to their constituencies. However, when asked, none would refrain from engaging again. Their motivation stemmed from a deep disgust with the status quo and a conviction that they were called to do something beyond their own imagination. That was fuelled by personal experiences of transformation and from witnessing how diversity can be an asset and a source of creativity.

Personally, this process of inquiry has taken me on an extremely interesting, challenging and rewarding leadership journey. When facilitating cross-sectoral processes in the described manner, one needs to hold up a mirror and reflect on one's own actions consistently. Consequently the journey has not only been outwards, but also inwards. It challenged me to examine my thought processes, my emotional intelligence and my intentions. As a consequence, I had to adjust my own way of operating. I started looking at my team, the organisation and its interactions with partners in a different manner.

Notes

1. The price of antiretrovirals reduced by about 54% in Latin America and the Caribbean Islands in 2002–3 (Henderson 2002).
2. The approach was relatively new in the social field as was its philosophy to adapt to local circumstances continuously. Hence, no blueprint for such initiatives existed.
3. Sensing: 'The view from within – when seeing and perception begin to happen from the field. When you enter the state of sensing, you experience a collapse of boundary between observer and observed' (Scharmer 2007: 469).

References

Blair, D. 2005. 'Mandela: My Son Has Died of AIDS'. *Telegraph*, 7 January. Available at www.telegraph.co.uk/news/worldnews/africaandindianocean/southafrica/1480648/Mandela-My-son-has-died-of-Aids.html.

Henderson, C. 2002. *AIDS Weekly*, August. Available at www.aegis.com/pubs/aidswkly/2002/AW020806.html.

Hunter, S. 2004. *Black Death: AIDS in Africa*. New York: Palgrave Macmillan.

Kalungu-Banda, M., J. Flick and C. Scharmer. 2007. *Cross-Sectoral Leadership for Collective Action on HIV/AIDS: Discovering Common Purpose and Intent amongst the Guardians*. Chaminuca: Oxfam Southern Africa.

Kirungi, F. 2001. 'Uganda Beating Back AIDS: Leadership, Education and Openness Are Key to Progress'. *African Recovery* 15: 1–2.

Scharmer, C. 2007. *Theory U: Leading from the Future as it Emerges: The Social Technology of Presencing*. Cambridge: Society for Organizational Learning.

———. 2008. 'Executive Summary: Theory U, Leading from the Future as it Emerges: The Social Technology of Presencing'. Available at www.otto.scharmer.com.

Senge, P. 1999. *The Fifth Discipline: The Art and Practice of the Learning Organization*. Johannesburg: Random House.

Senge, P., C. Scharmer, J. Jaworski and B. Flowers. 2004. *Presence: Human Purpose and the Field of the Future*. Cambridge: Society for Organizational Learning.

Sydney Morning Herald. 2004. 'Mbeki Lashes Whites over Sexual Caricatures of Blacks'. 27 October. Available at www.smh.com.au/articles/2004/10/26/1098667767751.html.

UNAIDS (Joint United Nations Programme on HIV/AIDS). 2008. *Report on the Global AIDS Epidemic*. Geneva: UNAIDS.

Wheatley, M. 2007. *Finding our Way: Leadership for an Uncertain Time*. San Francisco: Berrett-Koehler.

3

Assertive Leadership Response to HIV and AIDS

The Moroccan Example

Fatima Harrak

This chapter presents an example of a successful leadership response to HIV/AIDS on the African continent. This success, in Morocco, was based on a strategy first formulated in 1986, which has since been refined three times; first, in 2002 through the formulation of a 'National Strategic Plan to fight HIV/AIDS 2002–2005' (NSP); subsequently, through the second NSP for the period 2007–11; and, most recently, via a third NSP for 2012–16, which was prepared and ready for implementation in 2011. The first plan sought to change the dynamics of HIV transmission by reducing risk, exposure and consequence. The success of its diverse programme (work with sex workers and clients, prisoners, drug users, women and young people) paved the way for the current NSP. A common feature of Morocco's response to HIV/AIDS, ever since creation of the National AIDS Control Programme in 1986, has been a society-wide focus. This chapter describes how the government strategy in Morocco evolved and the role of the political authorities in containing the epidemic.[1]

A brief history

Statistics from 2009 suggest that HIV/AIDS prevalence in Morocco is low at only 0.1%, which translates to 22 700 people in a population of

30 million in 2009 (Thorne 2009).[2] There are no precise figures for HIV/AIDS incidence. However, a total of 2 306 new cases were recorded between 1986 and June 2007; 1 568 (68%) of which were amongst people aged between 15 and 39 years old. In view of the high level of sexually transmitted infections (STIs) among the general population, the government declared Morocco a 'high-risk' country in 1986. The introduction of annual sentinel surveillance surveys in 1993 has enabled scientists to identify some patterns of HIV transmission in the country. Methods of identification included notification by medical professionals of STI or HIV cases, scrutiny of blood donations and follow-up on HIV infections.[3]

Indications of new patterns of prostitution and migration, both transnational and rural-to-urban, were seen as linked in some way to the rise of tourism, which was perceived to be a major factor in the rise of HIV infections. Changes in lifestyle and sexual behaviour were also noted as possible causes for the increase in the rate of infection. For instance, heterosexual transmission, both within and outside of marriage, accounted for about 24% of infections between 1986 and 2000 and 85% of infections between 2000 and 2005. The intimation was that HIV transmission was no longer primarily between men who had sex with other men.[4] A disturbing feature of the changing nature of the epidemic is increasing HIV prevalence amongst women. The proportion of women with HIV/AIDS compared to men rose from 16% in 1990 to 38% in 2000, then to 40% in 2005, in spite of overt government efforts since the inception of the National AIDS Control Programme in 1986. This is a major cause for concern among policy-makers because Moroccan women constitute the majority of citizens who are illiterate (or have minimal literacy skills) and have limited access to service, care and decision-making processes.

In the 1990s, foreigners – tourists and immigrants – accounted for a significant number of HIV and AIDS cases in Morocco. By 2007, however, 95% of the recorded cases were amongst the indigenous population. Prostitution, heterosexual and homosexual, had become more widespread and more visible with the growth of tourism and immigration. For instance, statistics released by the United Nations in

November 2007 estimated that the number of infected persons rose from 18 000 in 2006 to 20 000 in 2007, of which 90% were in urban areas and 52% in the environs of Agadir, Casablanca and Marrakech, which are Morocco's major tourist centres (Binoual 2007). However, there was also awareness that the changes in citizens' sexual behaviour might be a factor: a 2006 report by the Directorate of Epidemiology in the Ministry of Health found that among women infected with HIV in 2005 only 2.4% were working in the sex industry.[5]

In 2002, Morocco revised its strategy and formulated a 'National Strategic Plan 2002–2005', the implementation of which was funded by The Global Fund to Fight AIDS, Tuberculosis and Malaria (GFATM). The goal of the plan was to contain the HIV epidemic at the estimated general HIV prevalence rate of 0.15% and STIs at 0.16% of the total population. Specific objectives of the plan included:

- The reduction of vulnerability of the groups most exposed to HIV/AIDS infection in the priority action regions;
- The implementation of a social communication programme for the benefit of young people and women;
- The provision for the diagnosis and treatment of persons living with HIV/AIDS, including antiretrovirals (ARVs).

In 2006, Morocco's Country Co-ordinating Mechanism (CCM) reported on the achievement of the objectives of the first plan. Notably, in its introduction of the 2007–11 NSP, the CCM outlined the activities that had occurred in the fields of prevention, care, support and treatment and acknowledged the comprehensive reviews of the epidemiological and socio-economic conditions of the epidemic as well as the strong commitment and enduring leadership of the national political authorities (UNAIDS 2009). The nature and manifestation of this leadership in Morocco form the thrust of the discussion that follows here.

Engagement of national authorities

The king, and the royal family in general, has been at the forefront of Morocco's response to HIV and AIDS. On numerous occasions, King Mohammed VI has affirmed Morocco's commitment to addressing the epidemic effectively. He inaugurated HIV-testing and care centres and, together with his wife, Lalla Salma, visited AIDS patients across the country to help reduce the stigma associated with HIV infection. From the inception of the NSP, he has strongly supported comprehensive and multisectoral measures on AIDS:

> Morocco established an integrated and comprehensive strategy to fight AIDS. It consists of several actions including voluntary counselling and testing, and provision of anti-retroviral treatment (ARV) to all eligible patients. It involves all governmental entities and, most importantly, nongovernmental organizations and civil society in the awareness campaign implemented by the media and targeting young people and vulnerable groups.[6]

The queen attended the international conference of the 'First Ladies of Africa on AIDS', which convened in New York City in June 2005. In December 2007, the king's aunt, Princess Lalla Amina, who is also honorary president of the Pan-African Organization against AIDS (OPALS), called for a 'large-scale AIDS prevention campaign based on a participatory approach to generalize screening centres for high-risk populations'.[7] She also advocated for a better use of media resources in targeting young people in the AIDS struggle.

The national campaign has also benefited from the active involvement of government, led by the prime minister with the participation of seven key ministries: Health, Communication, National Education, Youth and Women Affairs, Armed Forces Health Service at the Ministry of Defence, Islamic Affairs and the Penal Division of the Ministry of Justice. The Ministry of Health, through its network of hospitals, health centres, training capacity and qualified personnel, is central to all the actions mounted by the government. It also allocates an annual budget for its national AIDS programme. The CCM, under the auspices of the Ministry of Health, articulates the strategy for fighting AIDS, raises the necessary funds for its execution and ensures comprehensive and timely monitoring and evaluation of programmes. Members of the CCM include representatives of academic institutions, multilateral and bilateral partners, community-based organisations, international non-governmental organisations (NGOs), including the Joint United Nations Programme on HIV/AIDS (UNAIDS) and the private sector. This group constitutes the national co-ordinating body for all AIDS-related funds and is entrusted with all the processes to ensure accountability. It is also responsible for harmonising monitoring and evaluation of all donor-funded national programmes.

Within the CCM, governmental actors intervene at different levels: Communication, in the media campaigns; Education, in curriculum development; Youth, Justice and Defence, in the establishment of HIV/AIDS programmes that target these high-risk populations; and Islamic Affairs, in the mobilisation of their religious personnel, particularly imams, for the education of the larger population. Through multilateral and bilateral co-operation, international organisations provide funds and conduct orientation and awareness programmes. The private sector intervention occurs mainly in the areas of funding and awareness campaigns targeted at the working class. Local and international NGOs represent the bulk of the expertise required for the implementation of, specifically, the prevention and care aspects of the programme.

Making prevention possible through communication

Communication has been integral to Morocco's HIV/AIDS campaigns. This has been principally driven by the Ministry of Communication, with substantial support and parallel campaigns by some members of the CCM. For instance, the minister of Health has broken the social taboo on open discussion of sex and sexuality through discussions and interviews on television and the radio. All efforts acknowledged the importance of effective communication to raise awareness among the population, to inform people about the channels and locations of available support and treatment, and to bring the vulnerable population to testing and care centres.

A major communication campaign endeavour occurred with the inauguration of the charter of the 'Media Initiative against AIDS' in 2004, which was jointly signed by the Ministry of Health, the Ministry of Communication, Moroccan radio and television networks and the

Federation of Newspaper Editors. In addition, the Ministry of Islamic Affairs facilitated interaction with religious leaders to gain their support and active involvement in raising awareness and knowledge of HIV/AIDS.

The multimedia communication strategy (TV, radio, press and outdoor media) was planned in four phases: the first phase was directed at raising awareness of the disease and infection hazards; the second phase for transmission modes and prevention means; the third phase focused on fighting stigmatisation and discrimination; and all these steps led to the final phase when people were encouraged to participate in anonymous screening. In addition a mobile unit travelled 4 000 kilometres across the country to provide information on HIV/AIDS to otherwise inaccessible populations.

Table 3.1:   Summary of public features of the campaign in 2004.

Media coverage in 2004	
National television airtime	308
Radio spots	450
Press releases	100
Billboards	125

In 2006, the campaign was expanded by 1 320 TV and radio adverts, 100 newspaper announcements, 200 posters in urban areas and a mobile stand roaming the country. During the summer months, the Ministry of Youth, in collaboration with the Association de Lutte contre le SIDA/Association for the Fight against AIDS (ALCS) and the United Nations Population Fund (UNFPA), organised a 'caravan'. The caravan consisted of teams of young volunteers who travelled with a van fully equipped with information and testing materials, supported by health professionals and communications specialists. The caravan parked at some of Morocco's most popular resorts on the Atlantic and Mediterranean coasts and also in the remote Atlas Mountains. The caravan visited nineteen youth campsites where more than 7 000 young men and women stayed and in less than a month, it was able to distribute 35 000 flyers and 15 000 condoms to young people and give 700 confidential and free HIV tests and voluntary counselling. Various other communication ventures were established within the framework of this multimedia campaign, namely peer education, theatre, CD-ROM, news-stands at markets, sports and cultural events and literary sessions.

Another innovation in the field of social communication was the Ensemble contre le SIDA/Collective against AIDS (SIDACTION). In December 2005, under the patronage of King Mohammed VI, the ALCS and the television channel 2M organised a telethon to raise funds for HIV/AIDS programmes in Morocco. This programme, aired also by the channel TVM1 with the animated characters of TV stars, such as Choumicha and Ali Baddou, had unprecedented audience ratings. Numerous artists and stars, from sports to cinema, took part in the programme and largely contributed to its success. Moroccan and foreign experts were also invited to comment on all issues relating to HIV/AIDS. The testimony of an HIV-positive person, Fatema, helped Moroccans give a human face to this epidemic and bolster the struggle against it. During the evening, 400 000 calls were made to the free green-line provided by MarocTelecom and donations were also collected. The event raised the equivalent of US$27 288.20 (236 000DH), of which 50% was earmarked for prevention and 47% to treatment. The best indicator of success of this operation, however, is the number of people who volunteered for free testing after SIDACTION, which has subsequently been multiplied by five.[8]

This same high level support is now regularly extended to national and regional festivals and popular celebrations, such as the Gnaoua Festival of Essaouira and the Jazz Festival of Tangiers, where NGOs and young volunteers organise awareness campaigns in the form of information stands, dissemination of HIV-prevention messages and distribution of condoms among young people and sex workers.

Another initiative of the ALCS was the 'National Testing Days' campaign, organised on 5–7 January 2007. The Olympic champion, Nawal al-Mutawakkil (now minister of Sports and Youth) and the popular comedian, Rachid El Ouali (who offered to be tested for HIV/AIDS publicly) launched the event. It was held in 37 cities and towns and resulted in the testing of 7 492 people in three days, an improvement on 6 401 tests for the entire 2005 calendar year. This increase in participation demonstrated the efficiency of communication through role models and leaders of opinion in breaking the taboo around HIV/AIDS and encouraging people to test and learn more about the disease.

Fighting stigma
Prejudice and social taboos in Moroccan Muslim society were a known constraint on initial HIV/AIDS interventions. Strong leadership, spearheaded by the king, helped to promote collective action against the social stigma surrounding HIV/AIDS. The Moroccan leadership seems to have realised that this was a prerequisite to any effort directed at reducing risky behaviours, mobilising care and support for those infected by the virus and diminishing vulnerability among targeted segments of society.

To maintain the integrity of the media messages and the stability of the state, the organisers expunged any offensive or misleading concepts but gave sufficient facts about the disease in order to reach the targeted public through the national and long-term campaign. This campaign used themes, slogans, keywords and images that sent pungent messages, which were comprehensible to the Moroccan population.

Religious leaders have been vital to Morocco's campaigns. In the Muslim context, religious scholars and imams were deemed to be key actors in fighting stigma and raising awareness. Through their weekly sermons and consultations on HIV/AIDS, along with distribution of information leaflets and even condoms to the young, they have contributed to improving the public's understanding of HIV/AIDS and helped to create a supportive environment for those infected and affected by the disease. That is why partnership with the Moroccan Ministry of Endowment and Islamic Affairs is central to the country's NSPs. In addition, the Ministry of Education introduced sex education into the curriculum and a wide network for the distribution of information material in the teaching establishments.

Business leadership was invited to participate in this campaign upon the realisation that AIDS was a potential threat to the financial and economic sector. Its response came in the form of not only financial resources but also in the provision of information about HIV and STIs in the working environment.

Celebrities in sports and the creative arts were also key actors in this campaign; their participation was crucial in influencing the perceptions and attitudes of the wide media audience, particularly the youth. They did this either personally, when called upon to give a hand in a specific campaign, or through their affiliation with NGOs. Their participation in the 'Summer Caravans', the 'National Testing Days' and other events targeting the youth has been decisive in the success of these operations.

A notable outcome was that in April 2006, Moroccans living with HIV created their own association, Annahar. Through this structure and through their membership of the CCM, they became involved in the development and implementation of HIV programmes.

Testing and counselling

In order to contain the spread of HIV the government entrenched some critical objectives in the NSP with a view to carrying out anonymous screening. Initially focused on the most vulnerable groups and some targeted regions, the need then arose to expand the voluntary counselling and testing (VCT) programme to the whole country. The Moroccan government went into partnership with the private sector to create an enabling environment for the successful implementation of the VCT programme. Facilities included those of the Institut Pasteur, the National Institute of Hygiene, private laboratories and hospitals, and health centres throughout the country. In 2002 the government established special HIV Advice and Test Centres, in addition to the existing facilities. These centres were exclusively run by NGOs because they could intervene in specialised areas, for example, in programmes relating to sex workers and homosexuals.

By 2004, 37 urban and rural HIV Advice and Test Centres had been created. Organisations involved in managing these centres included OPALS, ALCS, Ligue Marocaine de Lutte contre les MST/ Moroccan League for the Fight against STIs (LM-MST), Association Marocaine des Jeunes contre le SIDA/Moroccan Association of the Youth against AIDS (AMJCS), Association Marocaine de Solidarité et de Développement/Moroccan Association of Solidarity and Development (AMSED), the Association of Family Planning and the Red Crescent. Partly funded by GFATM, these centres provide free and anonymous counselling and testing, free ARV drugs and monitoring of all voluntary patients eligible for treatment. Some of these centres, which initially focused on sex workers, have trained the latter to teach their peers about HIV prevention and also to be distributors of condoms to women.

In 2004, the CCM discovered during an evaluation exercise that it had met and exceeded all its key objectives: nearly two million condoms were distributed in the targeted areas, 172 000 young people and women participated in HIV/AIDS awareness-raising events, 27 800 people benefited from education initiatives and 2 200 commercial sex workers and working women participated in the outreach activities. Moreover, a total of 1 120 peer educators were trained to support vulnerable groups, including working women, sex workers and young people, both in and out of educational settings.

As more health structures were established by the state, more HIV Advice and Test Centres were created. However, the introduction of mobile testing centres (some of which have been offered to neighbouring countries by King Mohammed VI) accelerated the pace of testing by considerably increasing access of the Moroccan population to free and anonymous testing. The number of people who were tested rose from 3 300 in 2003 to 6 000 tests in 2004, to 9 000 in 2005.

The NSP for 2007–11 built on these achievements and objectives; for instance, the aim was that by the end of 2011, the prevention programme should reach and influence one million people, have tested 150 000 more people and offer high-quality treatment and psychological care to 4 000 people.

Adapting intervention to reality on the ground
The Ministry of Health is the central agency for ensuring that Morocco's national response relies on evidence-based research. A key feature of the government's strategy has been regular review of its prevention and treatment programmes. For example, in collaboration with national, international, public and private partners, the CCM commissioned reviews in 2002, in 2004 and again in 2006, as part of preparing and evaluating the country's NSPs and funding proposals.

The Ministry of Health continues to take responsibility for the financing of ARVs and for providing the equipment and agents for the biological monitoring of HIV patients. It does this by relying essentially on state funding with a complementary contribution from bilateral, multilateral or international co-operative agreements. However, as mentioned earlier, NGOs have played a major role in screening and testing, prevention, social communication, support of people living with HIV and, particularly since the commencement the provision of triple therapy for all AIDS patients in 2003, in providing follow-up therapy.

The role of civil society
Civil society in Morocco became involved in facing the threat posed by HIV/AIDS relatively quickly, through the formation of the ALCS in 1988. This was the first initiative of its kind in North Africa and the Arab world and the ALCS now has eleven branches throughout Morocco. In the wake of this initiative other associations came into being, particularly after the International Conference on AIDS in Africa held in Marrakech in 1993. Because Morocco is a low-prevalence country, until 1997, most of the government's actions in managing HIV/AIDS were limited to prevention, which entailed providing information to the populations identified as 'high-risk' groups: professional and occasional sex workers, homosexuals and the prison population, in particular. The ALCS and, subsequently OPALS, played an important role in devising ethically sound methods to reach high-risk groups, in addition to advocating for the introduction of ARV therapy.

The introduction of triple therapy in 1990 and the partnership between the government and the private sector helped ultimately to reduce the cost of AIDS-related drugs by 40%. This process began in 2002 with UNAIDS' 'Drug Access Initiative', which was followed by the introduction of generic medicines in 2004 and, thereafter, removal of taxes and customs duties on HIV medicine. Today, the monthly cost per patient for ARV treatment is 500DH – (US$62) compared to 800DH (US$100) in 2004 and 13 000DH (US$162.50) in 1998.

AMSED was significant in advocating for national campaigns to include a focus on changing attitudes and behaviour, rather than only raising awareness of the danger of HIV/AIDS. One outcome was that the Ministry of Education integrated sexual education into the national school curriculum and HIV/AIDS became a component of its literacy programmes.

There have also been two important associated initiatives since 2004, both of which have been under the personal leadership of the king. The National Initiative for Human Development (INDH) was launched in 2004 as a strategy to fight poverty, marginalisation and insecurity among vulnerable populations (the poor, those in rural areas and slums, the handicapped and the homeless). A national plan for children was initiated in 2005 as an integrated strategy to improve child welfare and incorporates a chapter on HIV/AIDS directed to 'street or homeless' children.

Partnerships

Created for the purpose of developing a proposal to obtain GFATM financial support for Morocco's NSP, the CCM has been central to the development of a co-ordinated, multisectoral response to HIV/AIDS. Initially, the CCM consisted of representatives of the Ministry of Health and some other social ministries, UNAIDS representatives and civil society organisations (CSOs). Since its inauguration in 2003, the CCM has supervised the progress of the national response, has validated the country's contractual commitments and reports and designed sub-technical committees to work on different features of the response.

In 2004, following an evaluation of the NSP, the Ministry of Endowment and Islamic Affairs joined the CCM on a collaborative project to involve imams in HIV/AIDS initiatives. Furthermore, other new members were included. There were representatives from more government departments (Communication, Justice, Defence), from the private sector (pharmaceutical industry, General Confederation of Moroccan Enterprises, National General Practitioners Federation), from academia (Rabat and Casablanca Medical Schools and Hospitals, Higher Institute for Information and Communication) and additional CSOs (AMSED, AMJCS, National Medical Association, Red Crescent and Moroccan Association for Family Planning).

As a co-ordination authority the CCM brings together its partners regularly in plenary or committee sessions for preparing programmes, identifying priority proposals, monitoring programme implementation and co-ordinating reviews. The CCM thus constitutes a forum where the ethos is for each member to be treated equally and where problems are discussed openly for the purpose of reaching consensus solutions. This ethos of transparency is reflected in the website and forum of this institution where all the information concerning its composition, function, goals and various activities are exchanged freely and openly.[9]

Conclusion

The experience of Morocco described above illustrates that strong and collective political will is necessary for confronting HIV/AIDS. However, Morocco, like many developing African countries, has not reached the objective of universal access to prevention, treatment and care. The country is also still struggling with the rising social and gender inequalities that are a characteristic of the transmission of HIV in the country.

For Morocco, confronting HIV/AIDS has been deemed a national priority. A national plan for dealing with AIDS was established, which elaborated a concerted national strategy in a participative, decentralised, multidisciplinary and multisectoral way. The Moroccan case reflects assertive leadership within and across political and social authorities. Recently, UNAIDS recognised Morocco's success 'over the past few years, in asserting itself as a model for the Maghreb, Africa and the Middle-East in terms of progress made in the disease treatment and prevention'.[10]

Notes

1. This chapter draws on a number of official documents in French and Arabic that are not cited in the text but the list of references at the end of the chapter provides principal references for Morocco's national response to HIV/AIDS.
2. See statistics for HIV prevalence in Morocco at http://hivinsite.ucsf.edu/InSite?page=cr06-mo-00.
3. HIV prevalence was of the order of 0.16% among carriers of STIs in 2000, and in 2004, 600 000 new cases of STIs were registered over a period of one year (UNAIDS, UNESCO and WHO 2004: 3).
4. Sexual relations between men have always occurred in Moroccan society, but they are never discussed openly because of the prohibitions imposed by Islam and the national Constitution. However, such practices are now becoming more open, especially in major cities.
5. The same finding has been confirmed by the Pan-African Organization against AIDS (OPALS) in a study conducted in January 2008 in seven Moroccan cities. See UNAIDS (2009).
6. Extract from King Mohammed VI's speech at the United Nations General Assembly's Special Session on HIV/AIDS, New York, 25–27 June 2001.
7. See www.lematin.ma/Actualite/Journal/Article.asp?origine=jrn&idr=110&id=78148.
8. See http://data.unaids.org/pub/ArticleExcerpt/2006/20060404-uiamorocco_fr.pdf. SIDACTION is now a permanent programme of 2M.
9. See www.programmesida.org.ma/www.ccm.htm.
10. See www.maroc.ma/PortailInst/An/Actualites/UNAIDS+says+Morocco+a+model+in+terms+of+prevention.htm.

References

Alami, K. 2006. *Global Fund to Fight AIDS Tuberculosis and Malaria: Morocco Experience.* Rabat: Ministry of Health.

Benjelloun, S., S. Bahbouhi, A. Sekkat, N. Bennani, N. Hda and A. Benslimane. 1996. 'Anti-HCV Seroprevalence and Risk Factors of Hepatitis C Virus Infection in Moroccan Population Groups'. *ResVirol* 147(4): 247–55.

Binoual, I. 2007. '2000 New Cases of HIV/AIDS in Morocco in 2007'. *Magharebia*, November.

Boushaba, A., O. Awil, L. Imane and H. Himmich. 1999. 'Marginalization and Vulnerability: Male Sex Work in Morocco'. In P. Aggleton, ed. *Men Who Sell Sex: International Perspectives on Male Sex Work and AIDS*. Berkeley: University of California Press: 263–74.

Boushaba, A. and H. Hammich. 2000. 'Outreach-Based Prevention in Morocco among Men Involved in Sex Work'. In *UNAIDS Best Practice Digest*. Geneva: UNAIDS: 1–3.

Elharti, E., R. Elaouad, S. Amzazi, H. Himmich, Z. Elhachimi, C. Apetrei, J. Gluckman, F. Simon and A. Benjouad. 1997. 'HIV-1 Diversity in Morocco'. *AIDS* 11(14): 1 781–3.

Jenkins, C. and D. Robalino. 2003. *HIV/AIDS in the Middle East and North Africa: The Costs of Inaction*. Washington, DC: World Bank.

Mernissi, F. 1985. *Beyond the Veil*. London: Al Saqi Books.

Ministère de la Santé (Ministry of Health), Morocco. 2006. *Fighting Against AIDS in Morocco with the Global Fund Support*. Rabat: Ministry of Health.

Morocco National AIDS Program. 2001. 'Country Report'. Prepared for the WHO 11th Inter- Country Meeting of National AIDS and STD Program Managers, Casablanca.

Moussaoui, I. 2000. 'Preventing HIV/AIDS in Morocco'. *Voices from Africa* 10. Available at www.unngls.org/orf/documents/publications.en/voices.africa/number10/4moussaoui.htm.

Obermeyer, C. 2000. 'Sexuality in Morocco: Changing Context and Contested Domain'. *Culture, Health, and Sexuality* 2(3): 239–54.

Thorne, J. 2009. 'Morocco Facing up to the Reality of HIV/Aids'. *The National*, 5 March. Available at www.thenational.ae/news/world/africa/morocco-facing-up-to-the-reality-of-hiv-aids.

UNAIDS (Joint United Nations Programme on HIV/AIDS). 2001. 'Morocco Epidemiological Fact Sheet on HIV/AIDS and Sexually Transmitted Infections'. Geneva: UNAIDS.

————. 2009. 'Morocco: A National AIDS Response.' UNAIDS Best Practice Collection. Available at http://data.unaids.org/pub/Report/2008/jc1348_morocco_response_highlights_en.pdf.

UNAIDS, UNICEF (United Nations International Children's Emergency Fund) and WHO (World Health Organization). 2004. 'Epidemiological Fact Sheets on HIV/AIDS and Sexually Transmitted Infections'. Geneva: UNAIDS.

UNAIDS/WHO. 2000. 'Virginity and Patriarchy'. In P. Ilkkaracen, ed. *Women and Sexuality in Muslim Societies*. Istanbul: Women for Women's Human Rights/Kaddinin Insan Haklari Projesi: 203–14.

————. 2006. 'AIDS Epidemic Update'. Geneva: UNAIDS.

4

Socio-Economic Rights and Development

HIV/AIDS and Antiretroviral Service Delivery in South Africa

Shauna Mottiar

HIV/AIDS-related service delivery in South Africa is inextricably linked to socio-economic rights and development. Responses to HIV/AIDS have been guided by the constitutionally entrenched right to health as well as by the developmental mandate of local governments. These criteria have been challenged, however, by changing policies regarding HIV/AIDS, the role of the state in service provision, the way service users are viewed and ambiguities regarding the decentralisation of health services. Civil society service provision has culminated in innovative methods of maximising antiretroviral (ARV) therapy, which have yet to be engaged with and consolidated by various spheres of health provision. This step would further the delivery of services as being based on rights and in a way that would meet developmental goals.

The South African Constitution emphasises rights to service delivery with regard to housing, healthcare, food and water. However, the country continues to experience large-scale protests against poor service delivery and the performance of local government in general. During the 2004–5 financial year 6 000 protests were officially recorded and the numbers have been extraordinarily high ever since then (Delaney 2007).[1] The delivery of these essential services was originally the domain of the government's Reconstruction and Development Programme (RDP), formulated post-1994 to eradicate the injustices of apartheid and to realise the substantive democracy linked with development. However, this agenda was modified by the institution of a neo-liberal economic framework, the Growth, Employment and Redistribution (GEAR) policy, in the mid-1990s. The GEAR policy viewed development less as a task of the state and more as a task for non-governmental organisations (NGOs) and the private sector. More recently, there has been a significant rise in social expenditure and evidence of the government pursuing a more interventionist economic strategy in response to the national HIV/AIDS epidemic.

This chapter analyses HIV/AIDS service delivery in South Africa in relation to these policy changes and is divided into three sections. The first deals with South African services as rights and the role of the developmental state in enforcing these rights. The second section provides the context for HIV/AIDS-related services in South Africa through a discussion of how the state views service delivery and service users. The third section examines the roll-out of the public ARV programme in South Africa. This section highlights the challenges facing delivery of decentralised services in a way that meets developmental goals. It discusses the role of civil society in the roll-out of ARVs in South Africa.

Services, rights and the role of the state

> Everyone has the right to have access to adequate housing . . .
> Everyone has the right to have access to . . . health care services
> . . . and . . . sufficient food and water.
> *Constitution of the Republic of South Africa,* 1996

As the quote above makes clear, South Africa's Constitution safeguards socio-economic rights as well as civil and political rights. Ensuring realisation of these rights has, however, proved to be challenging. One statutory constraint is that the state is not obliged to act to enforce civil and political rights; it merely has to guard against violating them. They are also absolute and formulated with a high degree of precision so that courts can easily establish the obligations generated by them. Enforcement of socio-economic rights, however, requires action by the state but entails costs arising, for example, from increasing welfare provisions. Furthermore, these rights take time to be realised. Yet the connection between the right and the action may appear to be vague and so require more effort on the part of interested parties, particularly the judiciary, to translate and enforce them (De Vos 1997).

These difficulties were highlighted when five residents of an impoverished Johannesburg township, Phiri, challenged the City of Johannesburg's water-delivery policy. Their grievances centred on the prepaid method of delivering water services and the policy's restriction of free water provision to 6 000 litres per month (25 litres per person per day). The High Court judge ruled that the prepayment service was unconstitutional and ordered the metropolitan government to provide the residents of Phiri with the option of a metered supply of water. Furthermore, the judge ordered the government to increase its provision of free water to residents of Phiri to 50 litres per person per day (Liebenberg and Conteh 2008).

The Phiri case was significant because it departed from the principle of 'reasonableness' – consideration of circumstance and costs – used in previous Constitutional Court rulings with regard to socio-economic rights.[2] It embraced the notion of a minimum standard aligned to the vision of the Constitution to transform the nation. The judge observed:

> It is . . . common cause that in the present matter, the average household consists of minimum persons of 16. It is further common cause that it takes 10–12 litres to flush a toilet in water borne sanitation areas. It is also common cause that the residents of Phiri township are mainly poor, uneducated, elderly, sickly and ravaged by HIV/AIDS. Many of them survive on state pension or grants. In these circumstances, it is obvious that the 25 litres per person per day is insufficient for the residents of Phiri . . .

To expect the applicants to restrict their water usage to compromise their health by limiting the number of toilet flushes in order to save water, is to deny them the right to health and to lead a dignified lifestyle. It is common cause that the people suffering from HIV/AIDS need more water than those not afflicted by the illness. Such persons require water regularly to wash themselves, drink, wash their clothes and cook. Their caregivers are also constantly expected to wash their hands. In this context waterborne sanitation is a matter of life and death. In this context the 25 litres per person per day is woefully insufficient . . .

It is uncontested that the respondents (The City of Johannesburg, Johannesburg Water, The Minister of Water Affairs and Forestry) have the financial resources to increase the amount of water required by the applicants (five residents of Phiri) per person per day. It is common cause that the respondents have decided to rechannel the 25 litres per person per day supplied for free to households that can afford to pay for water. The share that the respondents are allocated by the Treasury, for the purposes of utilising towards the realisation of the provision of water, has not been utilised. The various policies adopted by the respondents such as the Special Cases Policy, the Indigent Persons Policy, the Social Package Proposals and the Mayoral Committee decision of October 2005 all point to one direction; the ability of the respondents to provide more water than 25 litres per person per day. It is undeniable that the applicants need more water than the 25 litres per person per day and that the respondents are able within their available resources to meet this need. The respondent's provision of 25 litres per person per day is unreasonable. It appears that they are able to provide 50 litres per person per day without restraining their capacity on water and their financial resources.[3]

What emanates from these observations is, first, an emphasis on how the poor and marginalised are not only entitled to basic services but require them to mitigate further deprivation. Second, the observations assert that human rights should inform the provision of basic services. Both points are pertinent in view of South Africa's constitutional, political and economic commitment to achieving substantive goals. By 'substantive', I mean that which promotes development – the process of expanding the real freedoms that people enjoy and removing the sources of 'unfreedom', such as poverty, poor economic opportunities, lack of public facilities and social care (Sen 1994: 4). The developmental state establishes social and economic goals with which to guide the process of development and social mobilisation. Development, therefore, incorporates the principle of sustainability in terms of managing the delicate balance between economic growth and social development (Fakir 2007). In other words, sustainability means moving beyond a narrow concern with economic growth and paying due attention to the quality of growth. This includes ensuring that people's basic needs are met and that cross-sectoral concerns are integrated into decision-making processes and that communities are empowered (Fitzgerald, Mclennan and Munslow 1995). However, subsequently, in 2009, the judgment was reversed in the Constitutional Court, highlighting the difficulties of interpretation and implementation of these principles.

The government's RDP promoted substantive democracy by seeking to to eradicate the inequalities of apartheid through the rapid delivery of social goods:

> The central objective of our RDP is to improve the quality of life of all South Africans, and in particular the most poor and marginalised sections of our communities. This objective should be realised through a process of empowerment which gives the poor control over their lives and increases their ability to mobilise sufficient development resources, including from the democratic government where necessary. The RDP reflects a commitment to grassroots, bottom-up development which is owned and driven by communities and their representative organisations.[4]

The intentions are expressed rhetorically in the phrase, 'A better life for all', used by the African National Congress (ANC) political party in its various electoral and public relations campaigns.

However, it has been argued that the logic and aims of the RDP were contradicted by the ANC-led government's adoption of the GEAR policy as a macroeconomic framework in 1996. The RDP stressed a leading role for the state in meeting basic needs, developing human resources and building the economy, the state and society in general. In contrast, the GEAR policy envisaged a greater role for NGOs, notably the private sector, in generating development while the government's primary role was to be a facilitator through exercising fiscal restraint and initiating budgetary reform and public sector asset restructuring (Bond 2000; Chipkin 2000: 57; Lodge 1999). Development, in terms of the GEAR policy, is not a matter of state investment in social welfare but of the government building appropriate alliances and partnerships with non-state agencies to deliver services. More recently, there have been indications that the government has revived the logic of the RDP in the form of marked increases in social expenditure and more direct intervention in the economy (Habib 2004).

The government's HIV/AIDS strategy initially rejected provision of treatment in favour of prevention of the spread of HIV. The government saw civil society being 'partners' in service delivery. Civil society organisations actually went further, advocating for government provision of ARV therapy and even initiating treatment programmes in different localities. Various policy documents affirmed the role of civil society even after the government changed its strategy and began to create a public ARV programme.

My interest is in the question of how far HIV/AIDS-related service delivery has affected the realisation of substantive democracy in South Africa in view of the relationship between the epidemic and poverty. A United Nations declaration on HIV/AIDS asserted: 'In many parts of the world the spread of HIV/AIDS is a cause and consequence of poverty'.[5] It has also been argued that for many people vulnerability to HIV is initiated and driven by external factors, such as inherited disadvantage together with political and economic policies that exacerbate inequality. Once the risk has translated into infection, however, actual poor health provides its own 'internal motor to the cycle of inequality' (Heywood 2008: 3). So, unless people have access to healthcare services, illness adds to pre-existing deprivation. Illness incapacitates people, creating new needs and diverting household resources; hence 'HIV infection becomes not just a symptom, but an agent of inequality'. Heywood has further argued that this 'agent' needs to be challenged on two levels: directly, through public health campaigns to diagnose, prevent and treat HIV, and politically, through challenges to the policies which create or fail to alleviate the risk.

Prevention is better than treatment: HIV/AIDS-related services 1994–2003

The government's HIV/AIDS policy has been the subject of much debate. The ANC placed the HIV/AIDS crisis on its agenda in 1991 before it officially came to power in 1994. The party's health secretariat and the apartheid government's Department of National Health and Population Development formed the National AIDS Committee of South Africa (NACOSA), which brought together political parties, trade unions, the business sector, civic associations, government departments, health workers and academics. Following the 1994 election, the country's president, Nelson Mandela, endorsed NACOSA's strategy for implementation via the Minister of Health, Nkosazana Dlamini-Zuma. By 1996, it had become clear that the government's response was failing. HIV prevalence levels had doubled from 7.6% in 1994 to 14.2% in 1996 (Van der Vliet 2004).

After the second general election in 1999 and under the helm of President Thabo Mbeki, the health portfolio was given to Manto Tshabalala-Msimang. In May 2000, the Department of Health initiated its *HIV/AIDS/STD Strategic Plan for South Africa 2000–2005* (Department of Health 2000). Missing from the Plan was any commitment on the part of the government to the treatment of HIV/AIDS. The Plan focused only on the prevention and management of HIV/AIDS, rather than on treatment for HIV-infected people. The government's stance was publicly contested by a civil society organisation, the Treatment Action Campaign (TAC), which took legal action over the government's refusal to make nevirapine available to HIV-positive pregnant women to prevent mother-to-child transmission. In July 2003, the government was compelled to provide treatment to pregnant mothers by the Constitutional Court, which held that the government had violated the constitutional right of citizens to good health.

The reasons behind the government's refusal to provide ARVs to HIV-infected South Africans are assessed in detail elsewhere (see, for example, Mbali 2004; Gumede 2005). The general argument is that the government's adoption of 'fiscal discipline' and a neo-liberal macroeconomic strategy, favouring privatisation of basic social services, reducing social spending and liberalising trade relations, hindered the formulation of substantive policies to address poverty and inequality. The government's strategic HIV/AIDS and sexually transmitted disease (STD) plan resulted, therefore, in only half a service being offered to South African citizens. In other words, those infected with HIV/AIDS were seen by the state, as less 'service providable' than those who were not, and rights to services seemed to apply primarily to those who could be prevented from being infected. The net effect, according to activists, was that approximately six hundred people were dying every day of AIDS-related illnesses (Achmat 2004).

A study conducted between 2002 and 2004 on HIV/AIDS and service delivery detailed the nature of services under the 2000–5 Plan (Blaauw et al. 2004).[6] The Constitution allocates health responsibilities to all three spheres of government – general health services are shared between national and provincial spheres and the local sphere is made responsible for municipal health services. The 2003 Health Bill, while tasking local government with direct responsibility only for environmental health, provided for additional functions to be delegated to competent municipalities. The study found that 'the Plan is mainly concerned with involving other departments and sectors in the campaign against HIV/AIDS' (Blaauw et al. 2004: ii). Despite the Plan being vague as to how the tasks would be allocated and co-ordinated, there was reasonable consensus among government respondents regarding the roles of different actors in implementing it. The Department of Health was seen as having a legitimate role in steering the HIV programme and providing conditional grants to provinces. The role of provincial departments of health was to modify national policies according to provincial realities and process funding to local levels, including to NGOs. Local health facilities were seen as having a role in the provision of clinic services, advocacy, training, home-based care and garnering NGO support. Hospitals and clinics were described as being responsible for clinical service provision – the treatment of STDs and opportunistic infections. NGOs were seen as legitimate and important HIV/AIDS actors in the provision of home-based care, education, counselling and training.

The primary goals of the 2000–5 Plan were to 'reduce the number of new HIV infections' and 'reduce the impact of HIV/AIDS on individuals, families and communities' (Blaauw et al. 2004: 16). The strategies would include education and communication strategies, increasing voluntary HIV testing and counselling, improving STD management and the treatment of opportunistic infections, promoting increased condom use and improving the care and treatment of HIV-positive people and people living with AIDS to promote a better quality of life (Department of Health 2000). National, provincial and local government officials interviewed in the 2004 study saw their function as trying to reduce the number of infections and prevalence by linking these elements with care and support, which would include treatment (presumably of STDs and opportunistic infections) (Blaauw et al. 2004: 29). A local official commented that partnerships were crucial in being able to make the difference in both prevention and management (30).

The Plan passed the responsibility for service delivery to stakeholders other than government. The reason for this, aside from government abdicating its mandate to provide services, may be because government is too far removed from the problem locality. A national official noted: 'Some of the weaknesses inherent in any national programme . . . [are] that you are slightly removed from the implementation level and essentially . . . you're creating guidelines and policies and standards for something you are not involved in every single day' (Blaauw et al. 2004: 30).

Table 4.1 Roles and responsibilities of the national, provincial and local departments of health.

Roles and Responsibilities	National Department of Health	Provincial Department of Health	Local Department of Health
Steering	• Leadership • Provide strategic direction • Policy development • Define norms & standards	• Adapt national policies programmes to provincial circumstances • Develop plans to operationalise policies and strategies	
Support	• Develop guidelines &protocols • Provide technical support to provinces • Training	• Provide appropriate environment for implementation • Training • Capacity development	• NGOs • Community-based organisations
Financing	• Mobilise resources • Allocate resources • Provide resources for national programmes (conditional grants) • Funding of NGOs	• Mobilise resources at provincial level • Allocate provincial resources	
Oversight	• Monitoring & evaluation		
Service provision		• Hospital services	• Implementation • Clinic services • Prevention
Co-ordination			• Serve as channel to communities • Integrate local level resources
Broader development			• Infrastructure • Poverty alleviation

Compiled from Blaauw et al. (2004: 35, 37, 38)

It is for this reason that processes of decentralisation begin to make sense with regard to delivering services relating to HIV/AIDS. This was acknowledged by two provincial HIV directors: 'Remember at national, services are not delivered. National is a policy making body and coming up with strategies. Provinces are the ones who have got to customize strategies and put in plans to operationalise these national strategies and policies' (Blaauw et al. 2004: 37). Furthermore:

> Even within the provinces local government is the sphere where service delivery actually takes place. If now we decide as the province that is our role, we can ask local government to implement it for us and we can use them as an agent to do that either by devolving the function to them or us, there's this thing delegation and assignment, so one can do that (Blaauw et al. 2004: 38).

The challenges to decentralisation regarding service delivery are, however, summed up by local government officials who cite the lack of finances, resources and opportunities to build local institutional capacity as impediments to delivery within the realm of HIV/AIDS-related services. A local government official made this clear:

> We have a limited budget . . . in our district we don't have a special allocation for HIV/AIDS programmes. We mainly depend on grants. There is a lot of red tape in accessing the budget . . . and we have limited resources . . . there is too much work placed on especially the nurses that are working at the facilities (Blaauw et al. 2004: 32).

A more critical local government health official argued that HIV/AIDS treatment and care had not been adequately mainstreamed into general patient care at hospitals and clinics. Furthermore, he asserted that while home-based care was an important advance it could be viewed as a cheap alternative to institutional care and was not receiving adequate resources in the HIV/AIDS programme. Another weak point mentioned was that relying on volunteers for voluntary counselling and testing meant the risk of losing skills and personnel when the volunteers left to take up paying jobs; hence, an opportunity to build institutional capacity was lost (Blaauw et al. 2004: 31).

Local government officials emphasised not only a role for local health in HIV/AIDS service delivery but also for local government in general:

> Well, apart from the obvious [roles] like primary health care and the running of home-based care programmes . . . I think in addressing the impact of AIDS on communities and in mobilising communities to firstly come up with programmes of their own to solve their own needs, but also to be able to support communities in addressing those needs. I'm thinking in particular in terms of orphans, nutrition, yes, home-based care which I have already mentioned, strategies to alleviate poverty, food production, all other issues that go around HIV and AIDS. The issue of help for traumatised women and rape victims, etc., that also relates to AIDS. I think those would be better run at local government level in a lot of areas. Certainly where there is local government with some capacity, I feel that they would have a useful role to play there. But on the whole, local government has been sidelined (Blaauw et al. 2004: 38).

Local government officials also claimed that they were strategically placed to be able to go into communities and conscientise people regarding attitudes, beliefs and information around HIV. This could lead to a mitigating of stigma and encouragement of HIV testing and counselling.

The importance of local government with regards to HIV/AIDS service delivery is borne out by the experiences of the 2000–5 Plan. Development can be well facilitated at local levels because of the proximity to the service users. If there is a need to strengthen, for example, a prevention of mother-to-child transmission programme in a district or local hospital, then local government is best situated to reflect on accessibility factors to the programme, such as the need for roads and transport. Providing the necessary roads or transport would be a way of reducing the sources of 'unfreedom' of HIV-positive pregnant women who could then access the prevention of mother-to-child transmission programme at the local clinic. The limited levels of decentralisation to local levels under the 2000–5 Plan have been justified by provincial and national officials on the grounds of ongoing internal transformation, uncertain dynamics between district and local councils and capacity constraints. A provincial official claimed:

> There is this concept of the devolution of services to local government. We haven't, as yet, implemented this concept. But, what I see, I would say, the impact would be . . . the local at this moment, they do not have capacity in terms of understanding the whole concept of the HIV/AIDS strategy. And the second thing is, I don't think they have the budget to deal with HIV. And then, capacity in terms of supporting coordinators. I think that will also be a problem because they themselves need to be capacitated (Blaauw et al. 2004: 45).

To which a local official responded:

> It depends how you define capacity of course. There is an argument that if these local governments are given the resources that they will have the capacity, that capacity relates to resources . . . One can support the development of capacity through transfer of resources, through allocation of funds, through skills transfer, through seconding staff or various measures to assist local government to develop capacity. But to say they don't have capacity, therefore they never will have capacity, therefore nothing should happen through them, is not addressing the problem – it's perpetuating it (Blaauw et al. 2004: 45).

Ambiguities about decentralised health services in relation to HIV/AIDS, therefore, existed well before the provision of ARVs.

A better life for all: Roll-out of ARVs, 2003–4

In August 2003, just before an election year, the government finally instructed the Department of Health to begin the immediate roll-out of ARVs in public hospitals across South Africa. This was to be guided by an operational plan for comprehensive HIV/AIDS care (Department of Health 2003). The eventual provision of treatment followed protracted criticism of the South African HIV/AIDS policy from the TAC, which argued that the struggle was about constitutional rights to life, dignity and equity – because endangered life without medicine is death, dying of HIV/AIDS is often an undignified death and it should not only be people with money who can afford to buy life.

The 2003 Plan pledged itself to the provision of 'comprehensive care and treatment for people living with HIV and AIDS' (Department of Health 2003: 13). It was to achieve this by establishing a minimum of one service point in every health district (district council or metropolitan council) in the country by the end of the first year of implementation. Access to treatment would be made available to patients at these service points accredited to provide ARVs. The indication for proceeding with treatment would depend upon clinical assessment and CD4 count. Accreditation would depend upon human resource and technical capacity.

The Plan also laid out its drug procurement and provision strategy. The government's budget included more than R1 billion for new health professionals, R1.6 billion for ARVs, R800 million for laboratory testing and more than R650 million for nutritional supplements and support. There would also be more than R750 million for upgrading healthcare systems and R300 million for new capital investments. The Plan envisaged treatment at two levels – the primary healthcare level and the district/regional hospital level. Primary healthcare clinics and community health centres would be the primary sites for diagnosis and routine follow-up of HIV-positive patients. These sites would also provide ARV-adherence monitoring and support, counselling and nutritional assistance. Patients meeting the criteria for ARVs, however, would be referred to district or regional hospitals where treatment would be initiated and stabilised and would include treatment protocols and training on side effects.

The ARV programme only began in April 2004 and was described as 'painfully slow' (Hodgson 2006). The Department of Health continued to emphasise that since there was no cure for HIV, a focus on prevention should remain paramount. Again, this view seemingly privileged prevention over other components of a comprehensive response. Indeed, according to statistics put forward by the AIDS Foundation of South Africa, by early 2005 only about 30 000 patients were receiving ARV treatment in the public sector.[7] In December 2005, the health minister stated that 'about 85,000 people had been initiated on treatment in the public health sector by September 2005' (Department of Health 2005). According to the TAC, by the end of 2005, 110 000 patients were receiving treatment in the public sector (TAC 2006). Deena Bosch of the AIDS Law Project in Cape Town indicates that the Department of Health claimed that by March 2006, 130 000 people were receiving treatment in the public sector.[8] KwaZulu-Natal – the province with the highest HIV/AIDS prevalence in the country – fell well short of its treatment goals as evidenced by detailed 2004 statistics. The province set a target of treating 20 000 patients by March 2005. By the end of 2004, however, it was only treating 3 247 adults and 167 children (Gedye, James and Lebea 2004). By October 2006, the government reported that 224 895 patients had been enrolled to receive ARVs through public health services in all districts and prisons.[9]

As detailed in Table 4.2, according to 2007–8 figures, there were 350 000 patients receiving ARVs in public healthcare facilities, while another 524 000 required treatment but were not receiving it. The 2008 South Africa progress report for the United Nations General Assembly Special Session (UNGASS) on HIV/AIDS claimed that in 2007, 889 000 people needed treatment and that 488 739 were enrolled in the ARV programme, while 371 731 were initiated on the programme.[10] A study prepared for the Congress of South African Trade Unions in 2008 estimated the number of people needing treatment to be 1.7 million, while placing the number of people actually being treated at 371 000 and the number of people newly initiated at 120 000.[11] It should be noted that the reliability of these statistics is questionable, given the lack of information about patients who are lost to follow-up, deregistered or who die following commencement on treatment (Booth and Heywood 2008).[12]

Table 4.2   Summary of HIV statistics for South Africa.

Description	Number	Date	Source
People with HIV (prevalence)	5.6 million	2008	ASSA (2005)
People with HIV	5.4 million	2006	Department of Health (2007)
People over the age of two with HIV	10.8%	2005	HSRC (2005)
Pregnant women with HIV	29.1%	2006	Department of Health
People enrolled in the public sector ARV programme	488 739	End of 2007	South African Report for UNGASS (2007)
People who have actually initiated ARV treatment in the public health system	371 731	End of 2007	South African Report for UNGASS (2007)
People on ARV treatment in the public health system	350 000	2008	Aspen Pharmacare estimate, as quoted in *Business Day* (2008)
People on treatment in the private health system	100 000	2007	Joint Civil Society Monitoring Forum (2007)
People requiring treatment but not receiving it	524 000	2008	ASSA (2003)

Source: www.tac.org.za, using ASSA
ASSA = Actuarial Society of South Africa; HSRC = Human Sciences Research Council; UNGASS = United Nations General Assembly Special Session

The 2003 Plan was followed by the *HIV and AIDS and STI Strategic Plan for South Africa 2007–2011* (Department of Health 2007). The new Plan estimated that 5.54 million people were living with HIV in South Africa (9). This translates to 18.8% of the adult population being affected; women disproportionately so (55% of HIV infections). The Plan engaged with some of the substantive issues regarding HIV/AIDS. It noted, for example, that there were geographic variations in HIV prevalence. For example, the Western Cape province had the lowest level of HIV infection in the country (15.7%, according to 2005 statistics) but two localities, Khayelitsha and Gugulethu/Nyanga, registered prevalence of 33% and 29% respectively. These variations substantiated an earlier Human Sciences Research Council household survey, which concluded that people living in rural and urban informal settlements were at the highest risk of HIV infection and AIDS.

In an assessment of the earlier strategic plan, the 2007–11 Plan found that there was a broadening of involvement of agencies beyond the health department, which led to the establishment and expansion of key programmes, such as health education, voluntary counselling and testing, prevention of mother-to-child transmission and ARV therapy. Collaboration between the public health sector and local community-based organisations (CBOs), NGOs and faith-based organisations, which had begun before the public provision of ARVs were thus acknowledged and their relevance sealed. Civil society's response to home-based care, support programmes for stigma, nutrition and psychological aspects of HIV and programmes to increase access to legal services were all realised as vital to the success of public health sector treatment in general.[13]

The civil society response to HIV/AIDS prevention and treatment services has been constituted largely under the auspices of the South African National AIDS Council (SANAC). SANAC was established as an independent body in 2000 but restructured in 2006 to 'make it more effective and accountable in overcoming the HIV and AIDS epidemic' (Versteeg and Maredi 2007). This followed criticism that SANAC was not genuinely representative of civil society and that its processes were erratic.[14] SANAC is a multisectoral partnership body comprised of top-level government representatives and elected civil society representatives from a wide range of sectors.[15] SANAC plays a management and advocacy role in strengthening mobilisation, monitoring and providing national oversight in response to HIV/AIDS. It is specifically tasked with advising government on HIV/AIDS-related policy, creating and strengthening partnerships for an expanded national response and mobilising resources for SANAC partnership activities.[16] With regard to service deliverers, the Plan noted that the implementation of programmes tended to be vertical and that there were serious capacity challenges in rural areas. With regard to service users, the Plan noted that stigma and discrimination levels were high and deterred the utilisation of certain services.

The 2007–11 Plan had two main objectives: to reduce the number of new HIV infections by 50% and to reduce the impact of HIV and AIDS on individuals, families, communities and society by expanding access to appropriate treatment, care and support to 80% of people diagnosed with HIV. It has sought to achieve these aims by interventions in key priority areas: prevention, treatment, care and support, human and legal rights and monitoring, research and surveillance. The main goal was to reduce HIV and AIDS morbidity and mortality as well as the socio-economic impacts by providing appropriate packages of treatment, care and support. This entailed an increase in voluntary counselling and promoting regular HIV testing, increasing the retention of adults and children on ARVs, ensuring the effective management of HIV and tuberculosis co-infection, strengthening the health system and removing barriers to access. It also included mitigation of the impacts of HIV/AIDS and creating an enabling social environment for care.

The Plan is laudable because it made a commitment to treating those afflicted with HIV/AIDS and recognised that HIV-positive people have a right to healthcare in public facilities. It has been implemented alongside an increase in government expenditure on HIV/AIDS interventions. However, there are indications that the Plan is not being carried out to limit the 'unfreedoms' of poor people, notwithstanding the claim that the government's response to HIV- and AIDS-related services are 'comprehensive and developmental'.[17] Furthermore, in cases where civil society organisations innovated services to facilitate development objectives, the government (at all levels) seems to be failing to engage with them in a way that is replicable and sustainable.

In an assessment of the roll-out in rural areas, Gaede comments: 'It is striking how many services in rural places in South Africa have managed to provide ARVs to an amazing number of people' (2006: 23). Booth and Heywood (2008: 15) concur with this view but point out that disparities in access to treatment remain. Gaede claims that in his study many of the participating sites showed high rates of initiation of ARV treatment and high adherence rates. He argues, however, that one of the major stumbling blocks was the accreditation process. The accreditation process involved detailing whether or not a facility had enough doctors and nurses on staff to manage ARV delivery, whether the facility had adequate laboratory facilities and drug storage facilities, whether the referral network was operational and whether the facility was able to deal with tracing and following up with patients (Bodibe 2004).

The accreditation process hindered the implementation of primary healthcare models of ARV delivery because of poor co-ordination between national, provincial and local processes. A Joint Civil Society Monitoring and Evaluation Forum in 2004 found that there was a great demand for treatment because of the late commencement of treatment programmes, which was due to failure to accredit sites and the difficulties people faced in reaching accredited sites.[18] Human resources shortages and access to general resources were also sources of frustration. Gaede (2006) further criticises the accredited ARV clinics for over-reliance on doctors to provide medication. He argues that this is unsustainable, especially in the light of the above-mentioned skills shortage. Rather than a doctor-centric model with a vertical ARV programme, he advocates for integration of the ARV programme into the existing primary healthcare services. In this model, patients are assessed, undergo adherence training and are initiated on ARVs at the peripheral clinics by doctors and nurses. This approach leads to significant improvement of support to clinics as laboratory services and doctors' visits to the clinics increase.

Ford et al. (2006) elaborate on these criticisms; pointing out that roll-out coverage was highly variable among provinces because of a shortage of healthcare workers. They argue that the greater proximity and acceptability of services at the clinic level would lead to a much faster enrolment of people on treatment and much better patient retention. They substantiate their argument by referring to a particularly successful ARV programme in Lusikisiki, in the Eastern Cape province. This programme was initiated and run by the NGO, Doctors without Borders/Médicins sans Frontières (MSF), before the national ARV programme was implemented. It was officially handed over to the public health services in 2006.

Lusikisiki is a poor, densely populated, rural area in the Eastern Cape province where 80% of the people live below the poverty line. It had 95% coverage of people needing ARVs in 2005 and only 2% of patients were lost to follow-up in the clinics, compared with 19% at the local government hospital. Furthermore, patients arriving at the clinics with HIV were far less sick than was previously the case; in the inception phase of the project, people were so sick that had to be carried to the clinic or arrived in wheelbarrows. In early 2004, 50% of patients at the hospital and 40% at clinics arrived with a CD4 count of less than 50, but by the end of 2005 this had dropped to 16% at both hospitals and clinics. This was because people were seeking treatment sooner, with better immune status, which made clinical management easier.

Ford et al. (2006) argue that the Lusikisiki model was successful because it utilised three approaches: decentralisation to primary healthcare, task shifting within services and the creation of human capacity to support the system. With regard to decentralisation, the MSF clinics provided ARVs from the moment an individual was registered as a patient. This was different to the public health programme, which involved individuals being assessed at the local hospital and then referred to a clinic. This procedure entailed shuttling of patients, prescriptions and laboratory results between the hospital and clinics. With regard to task shifting, people's use of the Lusikisiki clinic services nearly doubled, from 16 465 in April 2004 to 28 191 in April 2006, as a result of implementation of the public ARV programme but the number of professional nurses did not change (30). Through training, mentoring and supervision, the running of the ARV programme was delegated to primary healthcare nurses and community healthcare workers, rather than relying only on professional nurses and doctors.

With regard to developing human capacity, the ARV programme included the training of lay workers to support the operation of a clinic-based HIV/AIDS service (patient support, treatment preparedness, follow-up visits and adherence). 'Adherence counsellors', for example, worked closely with other community members and organisations (for example, volunteer workers; support groups; and the TAC). The function of adherence counsellors, however, has yet to be formally accommodated in the Department of Health programme.

The Lusikisiki model exemplifies how innovative HIV/AIDS services reduce some of the 'unfreedoms' experienced by poor people by enabling access to life-giving health services. A low 2% loss to follow-up at local clinics suggests that patients find it easier to access local clinics rather than district hospitals and so they are more likely to use the facilities and adhere to ARVs. Furthermore the Lusikisiki model's creative solutions to skills and human resource challenges deserve consideration. The training and successful deployment of 'adherence counsellors', for instance, suggests that individuals are comfortable with being counselled and guided by people from their communities. The achievement of 95% coverage of ARVs for 2005 is clear evidence that the MSF model worked.

Conclusion

An outstanding feature of the Lusikisiki model is the prominent role played by the MSF. The MSF initiated its programme 'to strengthen the primary healthcare response' (MSF 2006). There is no doubt that the MSF model for an ARV programme expands rights-based services and furthers development objectives. The Lusikisiki model was instituted during a period of government ambiguity towards what constituted HIV/AIDS-related service delivery and whether services should focus on prevention or treatment. The MSF showed that this was an irrelevant question. The state, given its mandate regarding socio-economic rights, has a distinct responsibility to provide HIV/AIDS-related services. The epidemic raises particular challenges for the sphere of local government, which has a 'developmental' agenda. In so far as HIV/AIDS has the potential to undermine development processes, as vulnerability to HIV infection is associated with inequality and unrealised human development, the rationale for local government to respond to HIV/AIDS is 'obvious' (Van Donk 2008: 245).[19]

Substantiating state responsibility for HIV/AIDS-related service delivery and people's rights requires building local institutional capacity to 'free' the poor. One of the ways in which this could be achieved is by acknowledging and replicating innovative methods of service provision that have already been established by civil society organisations.

Notes

1. In 2009, the Centre for Civil Society at the University of KwaZulu-Natal was recording three to five protests a day in the country.
2. See *Government of RSA and Others v Grootboom and Others*, 2000, BCLR 1169 CC.
3. *Mazibuko, Munyai, Makoatsane, Malekutu and Paki v The City of Johannesburg, Johannesburg Water Pty Ltd, The Minister of Water Affairs and Forestry*, in the High Court of South Africa (Witwatersrand Local Division), 06/13865, 30 April 2008, Sections 169, 179 and 181.
4. *The Reconstruction and Development Programme*, 1994, Section 2.2.3.
5. *United Nations General Assembly 60/262 Political Declaration on HIV/AIDS*, 15 June 2006 (13).
6. This study formed part of a larger research project exploring key issues in the decentralisation and devolution of health services. It investigated, among other things, the key tasks needed for HIV service provision and the official allocation of roles and responsibilities to different actors in the public health system. The study covered a broad national overview of HIV/AIDS activities in the national, provincial, and local spheres of government.
7. See www.aids.org.za.
8. Telephonic interview with Deena Bosch, 30 May 2006.
9. *Government's Programme of Action 2006, Social Cluster*, South African Government, February 2007. Available at www.info.gov.za/aboutgovt/poa/report/social.htm.

10. *Progress Report on Declaration of Commitment to HIV and AIDS, Republic of South Africa, Reporting Period January 2006 – December 2007*, prepared for United Nations General Assembly Special Session on HIV and AIDS, p. 28.
11. *Progress Report*, p. 16.
12. Available figures from Statistics South Africa show that in 2011 the total number of people in South Africa living with HIV/AIDS was 5.38 million and that by the end of 2010 the estimated number of adults receiving ARV treatment was 1 058 399. See www.statssa.gov.za/publications/P0302/P03022011.pdf.
13. *Progress Report*, p. 27.
14. 'World AIDS Day: Reflecting on the Civil Society Congress'. Available at www.sangonet.org.za.
15. 'Brief on South African National AIDS Council', June 2008. Available at www.sangonet.org.za. 'South African National AIDS Council'. Available at www.gov.za.
16. AIDS Foundation South Africa, www.aids.org.za.
17. *Progress Report*, p. 27.
18. Inaugural Launch of the Joint Civil Society Monitoring and Evaluation Forum of the Operational Plan for the Comprehensive HIV and AIDS Care, Management and Treatment for South Africa, 7 September 2004, Polokwane.
19. In April 2007 the Department for Provincial and Local Government launched the 'Framework for an Integrated Local Government Response to HIV and AIDS'. The document specifies the role of municipalities and provides guidance on their responses to HIV and AIDS within their existing mandates (see Department of Provincial and Local Government 2007).

References

Achmat, Z. 2004. 'The Treatment Action Campaign, HIV/AIDS and the Government', *Transformation* 54: 76–84.

Blaauw, D., L. Gilson, P. Modibha, E. Erasmus, G. Khumalo and H. Schneider. 2004. 'Governmental Relationships and HIV/AIDS Service Delivery'. Centre for Health Policy Report, School of Public Health, University of the Witwatersrand, Johannesburg.

Bodibe, K. 2004. 'Where is the ARV Roll-Out?' Centre for the Study of AIDS Report, University of Pretoria, Pretoria.

Bond, P. 2000. *Elite Transition: From Apartheid to Neoliberalism in South Africa*. Pietermaritzburg: University of Natal Press.

Booth, P. and M. Heywood. 2008. 'Making Progress against AIDS? The State of South Africa's Response to the HIV and TB Epidemics'. Paper prepared for the Congress of South African Trade Unions.

Chipkin, I. 2000. 'A Development Role for Local Government'. In S. Parnell, E. Pieterse, M. Swilling and M. Wooldridge (eds), *Democratising Local Government: The South African Experiment*. Cape Town: University of Cape Town Press: 57–79.

Delaney, S. 2007. 'Amandla! Protest in the New South Africa'. Freedom of Expression Institute, presentation, 15 May.

Department of Health. 2000. *HIV/AIDS/STD Strategic Plan for South Africa 2000–2005*. Pretoria: Department of Health.

———. 2003. *Operational Plan for Comprehensive HIV and AIDS Care, Management and Treatment for South Africa*. Pretoria: Department of Health.

———. 2005. 'Speech by Health Minister Dr Manto Tshabalala-Msimang at World AIDS Day National Event'. Durban, 1 December. Available at www.doh.gov.za/docs/sp/2005/sp1201.html.

———. 2007. *HIV and AIDS and STI Strategic Plan for South Africa 2007–2011*. Pretoria: Department of Health.

Department of Provincial and Local Government. 2007. 'Framework for an Integrated Local Government Response to HIV and AIDS'. Pretoria: Department of Provincial and Local Government.

De Vos, P. 1997. 'South Africa's 1996 Constitution'. *South African Journal on Human Rights* 13: 66–101.

Fakir, E. 2007. 'Public Service Delivery in a Democratic, Developmental State'. *Policy Issues and Actors* 20(3): 3.

Fitzgerald, P., A. Mclennan and B. Munslow (eds), 1995. *Managing Sustainable Development in South Africa*. Cape Town: Oxford University Press.

Ford, N., H. Reuter, M. Bedelu and H. Schneider. 2006. 'Sustainability of Long Term Treatment in a Rural District: The Lusikisiki Model of Decentralised HIV/AIDS Care'. *Southern African Journal of HIV Medicine* 7(4): 17–22.

Gaede, B. 2006. 'Rural ARV Provision: Policy Implications for Accelerated ARV Roll-Out'. *Southern African Journal of HIV Medicine* 7(4): 23–5.

Gedye, L., C. James and M. Lebea. 2004. 'Putting the Government's HIV/AIDS Plan to the Test'. *Mail & Guardian*, 30 November.

Gumede, W. 2005. *Thabo Mbeki and the Battle for the Soul of the ANC*. Cape Town: Zebra Press.

Habib, A. 2004. 'The Politics of Economic Policy Making: Substantive Uncertainty, Political Leverage and Human Development'. *Transformation* 56: 90–103.

Heywood, M. 2008. *Health and the Inequality of Poverty: Towards a Rights Based Convention on Global Health*. Johannesburg: AIDS Law Project.

Hodgson, I. 2006. 'Dazed and Confused: The Reality of AIDS Treatment in South Africa'. 11 January. Available at www.opendemocracy.net.

Liebenberg, S. and S. Conteh. 2008. 'First Major Test Case on the Right to Water in SA'. *Legal Brief*, 12 May. Available at www.legalbrief.co.za/article.php?story=20080512121231959.

Lodge, T. 1999. 'Policy Processes within the African National Congress and the Tripartite Alliance'. *Politikon* 26(1): 5-32.

Mbali, M. 2004. 'AIDS Discourses and the South African State: Government Denialism and Post Apartheid AIDS Policy Making'. *Transformation* 54: 104-22.

MSF (Médicins sans Frontières). 2006. 'Lusikisiki Celebrates 2,200 People on ARV Treatment at Handover Ceremony'. Available at www.msf.org.

Sen, A. 1994. *Development as Freedom*. Oxford: Oxford University Press.

TAC (Treatment Action Campaign). 2006. 'Resolutions of National Executive Committee (NEC) Meeting, Cape Town, 20-21 June 2006'. Available at www.tac.org.za.

Van der Vliet, V. 2004. 'South Africa Divided against AIDS: A Crisis of Leadership'. In K. Kauffman and D. Lindauer (eds), *AIDS and South Africa: The Social Expression of a Pandemic*. New York: Macmillan: 48-96.

Van Donk, M. 2008. 'The Implications of HIV/AIDS for Local Governance and Sustainable Municipal Service Delivery'. In M. Van Donk, M. Swilling, E. Pieterse and S. Parnell (eds), 2008. *Consolidating Developmental Local Government: Lessons from the South African Experience*. Cape Town: University of Cape Town Press: 245-63.

Versteeg, M. and M. Maredi. 2007. 'Decentralised Response to HIV and AIDS'. Local Government Bulletin. Pretoria: Centre for Municipal Research and Advice.

5

Confusing Public Health with Militant Nationalism

South Africa's AIDS Policy under Thabo Mbeki

John-Eudes Lengwe Kunda and Keyan Tomaselli

South Africa has represented the epitome of disastrous national responses to Africa's HIV/AIDS pandemic. It has, nonetheless, opened up the intricate workings of health systems, policy formulations and their implementation, including the influence of cultural scripts in medical discourse. This chapter is a critical appraisal of the ethos within the denialist agenda that marked Thabo Mbeki's tenure as South Africa's president. This ethos was a myopic counterbalancing of a 'resistance to imperialism' and an 'African Renaissance' philosophy. Mbeki's tenure was marked by a stagnant ideology, rather than the necessary reinvigoration of an African ethic to contain the HIV/AIDS epidemic. As Barnett and Whiteside put it:

> *Abantu abaafa!* – People are dying! People are dying. Children are being orphaned. The elderly are left uncared for. Already disgraceful poverty is made worse. HIV/AIDS marks exclusions that can be found not only across the gross geography of continents, but also in the more subtle geography of social networks and city blocks (2002: 7).

Here are some experiential narratives of HIV and AIDS that outline this 'subtle geography':

> For me, I noticed when I saw 'the father of my child' started getting sick, but he never went to test until he passed away. The state that he was in scared me and I decided to get tested and I went to the hospital and they transferred me to this clinic to get my treatment [Woman].
>
> I looked at myself . . . the problem I had is that if I die what's gonna happen to my son? Who's gonna be there for him? What . . . what . . . what is gonna happen? Whose gonna take care of him? Things like that [. . .] because of this feeling, I decided to test for AIDS [Woman].
>
> They are scared and they . . . start getting sick, you ask them what is wrong and they say it's a headache or a flu until they die. They never say its HIV and AIDS. Even their mothers hide it from the community but go around pointing fingers at another neighbor's child and saying 'they must show us how does a person with this disease look like.' While their child is sick and they never talk about it, when the child dies they are ashamed [Man].
>
> They are scared; the people here are not like the people in the townships. This is a rural community they would say they have better things to do [Man].[1]

People's fears about HIV/AIDS were matched in South Africa for much of this decade by the misgivings of the country's president, Thabo Mbeki, about scientific and medical knowledge on HIV/AIDS. In 2001, he expressed the following in a television interview:

> Interviewer: Would it not be an example; the president taking an HIV test?
> Mbeki: No, but it is setting an example within the context of a particular paradigm . . . So do I go down the street dispersing these pills, knowing from the best science that there are

consequences, that our health scientists do not know enough? Please stop politicising this question; let us deal with the science of it. The panel said one of the things we have to do is to determine the following: when we do an HIV test, what is the test testing? What is it measuring? So I go and do a test, I am confirming a particular paradigm, but it does not help in addressing this health need. Our focus must be how to improve the health of our people and that is what we are focused on.[2]

The president appealed to the common good in likening his position to safeguarding the lives of his people by rejecting the prevailing scientific paradigm that people were dying as a result of HIV infection. His views were immersed within his broader ideological encouragement of an 'African Renaissance', a philosophy that seeks to bring Afrocentric ethics to systems of governance and international relations (Liebenberg 1998; Makgoba 1999). The basic tenet of this African philosophy is *ubuntu* (as the ontological basis of a communitarian life), an ethic that recognises the interconnectedness of human experience and the indispensable co-dependence of human interaction.

The different discourses outlined above highlight the contradictions for which South Africa achieved global notoriety. From 1998 till 2008, when Mbeki was replaced as the country's president, public health debates revolved around his controversial views and how they subordinated the country's response to the HIV/AIDS epidemic to a personal ideology (see Baleta 2006; Butler 2005; Makgoba 2000; Schneider and Fassin 2002; Younde 2007; 'The Durban Declaration' 2000; 'Mbeki's Mistake' 2007; 'News in Brief' 2007; 'South Africa's AIDS Plan' 2007). Mbeki's position and influence was unlike some other leaders in sub-Saharan Africa whose responses have largely been lauded (Stoneburner and Low-Beer 2004; Wendo 2003; Younde 2007). Mbeki was a 'dissident' but, it must be understood, this was in the context of the experience of apartheid wherein public health had been used as a tool of oppression (Schneider and Fassin 2002; Younde 2007). Furthermore, in the early 2000s, the high cost of antiretroviral (ARV) medicines was a national cause of concern and entailed legal disputes with pharmaceutical companies to force a reduction in prices (Tucker and Makgoba 2008).

Mbeki's position amounted to ideological stagnation, an inability to generate or change one's condition, which, in this case was marked by resistance to perceived 'Western', 'colonial' political agendas on the one hand and, on the other hand, philosophical appeal to the renaissance of an 'African spirit'.[3] He withdrew from public debate on the matter of HIV/AIDS in the early 2000s but, as we will illustrate shortly, he continued to exercise enormous influence on the direction of the country's national response to the epidemic.[4]

This silent diplomacy is symptomatic of the polarisation that is inherent within South Africa's social, economic and political landscape due to a fragmented past that has left wounds that will take a long time to heal. There is room for progressive leadership in terms of the African Renaissance philosophy but it cannot be dependent on personal ideologies. The dangers are well known and South Africa's experience is not unique. The American government under President George Bush, it must be remembered, has been criticised on the same grounds. We refer to that government's promotion of abstinence campaigns and imposing funding conditions upon recipients, such as prohibiting abortion services and working with prostitutes, on the basis of the influence by and support of Christian organisations for that president's electoral campaign (Altman 2005; Das 2005; McClelland and Fine 2008; Milio 2005). The gist of this critique is that the HIV/AIDS pandemic requires an extraordinary response from society and, hence reinvigoration, even reinterpretation of its political traditions. In turn, this means African leaders who are not rooted in the past but who can face the unprecedented challenge of HIV/AIDS with a vital ethic and practice.

Contextualising the argument

The shrugging off of the oppressive apartheid system not only occasioned jubilations of freedom but also unveiled festering social, political and economic wounds enmeshed in colonial trauma (Colvin 2003). The political landscape was unique. The resistance philosophy of South Africa's African National Congress (ANC) was cosmetically integrationist and at the same time seeking to balance power and wealth for the liberation of the oppressed groups. President Mbeki's convoluted 'resistance/Renaissance' ideology articulated this agenda with profound effects on the country's public health interventions on HIV/AIDS. His agent was the minister of health from 1999 to 2008, Dr Tshabalala-Msimang.

As late as 2008, South Africans were being advised of the minister's agenda. On Sunday, 24 February, a media report cited her as saying 'No clinical trials for South African healers' (South African Press Association 2008). She admitted the necessity of clinical trials but alluded to them as 'Western' means of scientific investigations, thereby invoking a well-established political discourse of polarising such means against 'African science' – in this instance, a rejection of the scientific protocols for research on traditional healers' methods and medicines.[5] The minister had frequently spoken before in favour of 'traditional' approaches to HIV and AIDS treatment (Watson 2005) and labelled anything 'Western' as antithetical to African ways (Dwyer 2003). Lest it be presumed that such thinking had little effect in scientific circles, convoluted explanations had previously found their way into academic journals. For example, Bolognesi inadvertently articulated this thinking in writing: '[It is] as a result of this persistent denial, even at the highest government levels, that western medicine of predominantly White origin continues to be met with an element of suspicion by black patients and traditional healers' (2006: 626).

The minister's discourse was one of postcolonial nostalgia that pitted 'Africa' against the 'West' and, in line with Mbeki's resistance/ Renaissance ideology, represented herself as a victim of Western machinations (Sidley 2006). Her search for an African solution to HIV/ AIDS lay in her insistence on the use of herbal remedies as opposed to ARVs and, in the process, endorsed a popular discourse that the latter were a 'Western' tactic to poison 'African' people (Bolognesi 2006). Most infamously perhaps, she advocated the use of garlic and beetroot to treat infection (Baleta 2006; Cherry 2006).[6]

The minister enjoyed the president's support; her deputy-minister did not. When Tshabalala-Msimang fell ill, her deputy, Nozizwe Madlala-Routledge, was propelled to the forefront of explaining and projecting the government's health policies. Madlala-Routledge was critical of the government's policies but also walked a fine line between political allegiance and dissent. For instance, in a response to accusations that she had called on President Mbeki to take an HIV test, she stated:

> Although I encourage people to test so that they know their HIV status, I did not, as a matter of fact, call upon the President to conduct a public test as claimed by the reports. The journalist asked me if I thought it helped if people in leadership positions tested, to which I responded in the affirmative.
>
> This was in response to me taking a public HIV test as part of the *Sunday Times* campaign for South Africans to get tested. The main point I was making was to unite all South Africans behind this important campaign for testing, which forms part of the National Strategic Plan on HIV and AIDS and Sexually Transmitted Infections (STI) for South Africa and the Comprehensive Plan on HIV Management, Care and Treatment, adopted by Cabinet in December 2003.
>
> I wish to reiterate my commitment to the policy framework as agreed by Cabinet to ensure that the whole of government communicate a single, clear and consistent message on HIV and AIDS (Madlala-Routledge 2006).

Subsequently, she was fired, supposedly for an unauthorised official visit but in public opinion because of her opposition to the minister's perspectives on HIV/AIDS and for calling a national health emergency in view of high child mortality rates occurring at two Eastern Cape public hospitals.[7]

As we have indicated, the 'resistance' dimensions of Mbeki's ideology distorted the notion of public health as a common good and, inevitably, rejected efforts for collaboration and pragmatic action between the state and scientists to contain the epidemic (Cherry 2000; Nattrass 2006, 2007, 2008). The presidency represents matters of the nation but public health cannot be an area for experimentation for its own sake or for ideological and philosophical perambulations. The president's refusal to dispense with a 'resistance' mentality was not only counterproductive but left the majority of his electorate like sheep without a shepherd.

His advocacy of a Renaissance philosophy achieved even less. Collective wisdom is a central tenet of the spirit of the African Renaissance. The notion of a Renaissance promotes learning from current cultures within an African ethic. It is rooted in the ethic: 'I am because we are, and because we are therefore I am' (Mbiti 1990). It is an ethic that recognises the interconnectedness of the forces of life (vitalogy). It is expressed by the term *ubuntu*, which emphasises humane co-existence. This presupposes a web of relationships that supports everyone in the social system, except for witches and wizards who are perceived as threats to the social and spiritual order of the community.

This is the idea that Mbeki invoked. He called for community, using the poetics of being an African, his people having to grapple with hunger, disease and post-apartheid disillusionment. The *ubuntu* symbol is a powerful human-centred concept that calls for an empathic communitarian engagement in seeking solutions to problems. However, if this principle was so important to Mbeki, there are some vital questions to ask:

- Where was *ubuntu* when 4–5 million people were living with the virus and not receiving adequate care?
- Where was *ubuntu* when people were subjected to pseudo-scientific concoctions and denied life-saving drugs?
- Where was *ubuntu*, in a context where people living with HIV and AIDS were being told that their condition may be caused by a number of factors but they would benefit from eating garlic and beetroot?

In the name of the African Renaissance: The hypocrisy of an African response

Activists in South Africa and internationally repeatedly called on the government to engage with the problem of South Africa's rampant HIV/AIDS epidemic. However, our contention is that they misconceived the situation as a difference of medical and scientific positions. There has been no engagement with the discourse at the root of Mbeki's ideology which, in essence, is rebellion against perceived imperialist forces in the form of medical and pharmaceutical organisations that enslave Africans. However, this is a difficult terrain on which to engage Mbeki and those who subscribe to his views. To criticise Mbeki's ideology as a reactionary philosophy that cannot liberate oppressed Africans is to risk being labelled a traitor or a racist.

The desire to develop an African response to problems occurring in Africa is a legitimate agenda, even though 'African' is a contested concept (Mbigi 1995; Tomaselli 1999; Zeleza 2006). Nonetheless, in terms of *ubuntu*, some points are evident: it requires a definition of 'African' that moves beyond political categorisations of people on the basis of skin colour, embraces ethnic diversity and encourages an ethos of collectively negotiated worldviews. What is disturbing in the South African ethos, as represented by Mbeki's ideology, is that it amounts to a deep-seated suspicion of 'Western' societies as intrinsically oriented towards the manipulation and subjugation of 'black' Africa and, hence, emphasises reaction to the threat of recolonisation and resubjugation of the 'black' people. In contrast, 'African' in terms of *ubuntu* imagines solidarity within a web of shared communion. It means being with everyone within given spaces and using available resources for the pursuit of mutual benefit. Philosophically, *ubuntu* expresses a web or network of relationships. In an Afrocentric ethos, everyone within the network shares all that is life – sickness and pain as well as joy. However, Mbeki's ideology trivialises South Africans' pain and loss in poetic debates of whether there is a link between HIV and AIDS and death.

The people of South Africa are experiencing sickness and death on a vast scale irrespective of whether we know exactly the multiple links between the virus, opportunistic illness, the AIDS condition, poverty, inequalities and past and present social inequities. Listening to their stories reveals the extent to which Mbeki's discourse on the 'health of our people' is unconnected to their experiences and to their lives. Stories of ordinary people struggling with HIV and AIDS have been researched extensively (Campbell et al. 2005; Dorrington, Bradshaw and Budlender 2002; Dwyer 2003; loveLife 2001; Marais 2005). And yet, did the state's African Renaissance philosophy, as represented in Mbeki, listen to these stories of pain? Does this philosophy reveal care by the state during his tenure as president and integration of these individuals' experiences into government initiatives? How has the preoccupation with fighting imperialism and warding off re-enslavement helped the country to reduce people's suffering? Mbeki's ideology, ironically, represents disease as affecting others and, as such, is akin to the denials of HIV infection and AIDS deaths that can be heard regularly in this country's communities.

It will be noted that our questions above are polemical and deliberately so, as a means to uncover the nuanced hidden ideological agenda in public health policy and to demystify Mbeki's ethnic slant in his interpretation of the epidemic. The essence of our argument is that there is a close tie between political leadership and the fuelling of conspiracy theories. In public health policy, it is critical to recognise that the political voice is not only manifested in policy decisions and documents but also in the public utterances of leaders, which have ramifications for public discourse. We argue, as others have done, that the position of Mbeki fuelled and legitimised some of the existing conspiracy theories as well as fostering a climate of denial and ironically, stigma and discrimination (see Niehaus and Jonsson 2005). To illustrate, one media publication was headlined 'South Africa: AIDS Conspiracy Believers Less Likely to Condomise', indicating that denialism anchored in conspiracy theories has a correlation with behavioural patterns.[8]

Denialism has infected the South African public

Through popular discourse, individuals known to be HIV positive are ostracised and separated from their communal bonds. Kunda (2006) identifies a number of discourses that have emerged in reference to HIV and AIDS, in the area known as the Valley of a Thousands Hills outside Durban. Here, we discuss four popular discourses of denial.

First, a *cleansing discourse* distinguishes those who are and those who are not infected. Metaphors include 'Omo', a common brand of washing powder. Omo is likened to 'washing away' (of infected persons) and the removal of unwanted stains or dirt (infection) from clothes (society). 'Sieving' and 'winnowing' are other terms used in the same way; they describe removal of chaff (sick, infected persons) from grain (uninfected persons, the community) and, more abstractly, that which needs to be separated from what is essential.

Second, there is a *discourse of commonality*, which is invoked by reference to the word '*Ipot*', the term for the traditional three-legged pot used for cooking over a fire.[9] The pot is used in collective cooking activities. It is used in reference to HIV/AIDS, to indicate that something is 'boiling' or 'cooking' in someone's body. When the thing is brought to the boil, then the individual is ready for death and the metaphor is used to remind an infected person to prepare for his or her death.

Third, there is a *discourse of stigma*. Channel O, a risqué pop-music television programme is one metaphor used to connote sexual promiscuity as cause of infection as well as to indicate an infected person. Furthermore, a person who goes for voluntary testing and counselling is called a 'Channel O'.

Fourth, there is a *discourse of 'blame by association'*, which uses reference to 'BMW Z3' (or 'Z3'), an expensive sports car model, to summarise a number of linked judgements about people who return from life in the cities to die at their rural homes. The car, a symbol of wealth, also signifies the high life and fast living, with inferences of sexual promiscuity and the unsustainable nature of such a life, which leads to death. Ironically, it is also associated with the campaigns by loveLife, a non-governmental organisation (NGO) that has boldly promoted an aspirant, urban youth culture to cultivate self-interest amongst teenagers through its campaigns for safe sex and preventing HIV infection (see Chapter 10).

These are disturbing discourses, for they condemn those who are seen or are perceived to be ill as a result of HIV infection. These are not discourses that embody the principles of *ubuntu*. They are discourses that infer that HIV/AIDS is a foreign intrusion that threatens the social fabric of rural communities. The metaphors emphasise exclusion of those who are infected. They are discourses that accentuate individuals' fears. Narratives of people's experiences reveal deep despair when seen in this light:

> . . . fear of losing weight and showing signs that you are sick and the community seeing your body change and knowing that you have AIDS. You lose weight and it is over for you, the community starts to ask when . . . they say when is the funeral date . . .
>
> I never tried to test blood but I think it is right to continue. I am afraid to test because . . . they might find that I have HIV and people will look at me in a different way you see and [. . .] the community to know . . . because it happened in KwaMashu there is a girl who was known to have HIV and she was stoned to death . . . in other words . . . you are afraid of your life sometimes. You wish you can come . . . despite when you come but make it your secret (Kunda 2006).

When Mbeki chose the philosophy of an African Renaissance, he invoked a vision of humane co-existence. The strength of this vision is its communalistic ethos (Bujo 1990; Mbiti 1969; Moemeka 1998; Nyamiti 1989; Tempels 1959). The 'I' is intricately woven within the 'we'. The whole web is affected when individuals fall sick. No one exists save in communion with others; in other words, one's existence is owed to others (Mbigi 1995). It is an admirable philosophy but one which Mbeki has not applied to HIV/AIDS with the same vigour as he has applied his 'African resistance to imperialism' ethic. Espousing an African Renaissance at leaders' forums across the continent and further afield counts for nothing in view of the corruption of this cultural foundation of community life at home and by those who should and could be most supportive of it.

Conclusion
The state exists for the common good. Mbeki, during his tenure as president of the South Africa, established an intellectual and,

potentially, a popular agenda, which could have built upon Mandela's agenda of reconciliation. Instead, his 'resistance/Renaissance' ideology marked his stagnation as a leader. The African Renaissance philosophy deserves better cultivation, specifically:

- Transcendence of Mbeki's personal ideology that is anchored in diametric opposition of 'Western' and 'African' perspectives. There is space to learn from the best of both traditions;
- *Ubuntu*-centred public health is a commitment to collective, mutual support within which leadership expressed in the best efforts and thinking of scientists, NGOs and activists must be acknowledged;
- An unambiguous voice from the presidency in support of collective action.

For Africa, as elsewhere, times have changed. It is time for reinvigoration of the body politic.

Notes

1. These narratives come from a study conducted in a rural area of KwaZulu-Natal (Kunda 2006). They are excerpts from focus group discussions. The purpose of the study was to explore people's experiences of HIV and AIDS. All informants were members of a support group of people living with HIV and AIDS.
2. Transcription of e.tv interview with President Thabo Mbeki. Available at http://64.233.183.104/search?q=cache:L_Y8K6_DiCAJ:www.thepresidency.gov.za/main.asp%3Finclude%3Dpresident/interviews/2001/int0424.htm.
3. The 'African spirit' is an ideal rooted in a history of contradictions. There is no specific meaning to being African; representations differ in different discourses (Zeleza 2006).
4. AIDS was represented by Mbeki as a 'syndrome' rather than a disease, emphasising the viewpoint that people die of consequent opportunistic infections rather than of the disease itself (Nyonator et al. 2005).
5. Clinical trials are a method of investigation based on a philosophy of empirical research. They are a tool for the validation and or investigation of cases of public health concern (Braunholtz, Edwards and Lilford 2001; Oakley et al. 2006).
6. The minister seems to have been convinced by the claims of a self-proclaimed 'nutritionist', Tine van der Maas, who argues that taking a concoction of lemon,

olive oil, crushed garlic, spinach, ginger, beetroot and a solution of African potato would help in strengthening the immune system of AIDS patients (Deane 2005).

7. The public here refers to civil society as well as media as the arena of the interaction of the public and opinion is expressed in diverse arenas, not always easily referenced (see Geffen 2009).

8. See www.plusnews.org/report.aspx?ReportID=93042.

9. This is a contemporary word; the English word 'pot' is rendered into isiZulu by adding the Nguni prefix 'i'.

References

Altman, L.K. 2005. 'Study Challenges Abstinence as Crucial to AIDS Strategy'. *The New York Times*, 24 February. Available at www.nytimes.com/2005/02/24/national/24aids.html.

Baleta, A. 2006. '"Dr Beetroot" Sidelined in South Africa'. *Lancet* 6(10): 620.

Barnett, T. and A. Whiteside. 2002. *AIDS in the Twenty-First Century*. New York: Palgrave Macmillan.

Bolognesi, N. 2006. 'AIDS in Africa: A Question of Trust'. *Nature* 443(7112): 626-7.

Braunholtz, D.A., S.J.L. Edwards and R.J. Lilford. 2001. 'Are Randomized Clinical Trials Good for Us (in the Short Term)? Evidence for a "Trial Effect"'. *Journal of Clinical Epidemiology* 54: 217-24.

Bujo, B. 1990. *African Christian Morality at the Age of Inculturation*. Nairobi: St Pauls Publications Africa.

Butler, A. 2005. 'South Africa's HIV/AIDS Policy, 1994-2004: How Can It Be Explained?' *African Affairs* 104(417): 591-614.

Campbell, C., C.A. Foulis, S. Maimane and Z. Sibiya. 2005. '"I Have an Evil Child at My House": Stigma and HIV/AIDS Management in a South African Community'. *American Journal of Public Health* 95(5): 808-15.

Cherry, M. 2000. 'South Africa Turns to Research in the Hope of Settling AIDS Policy'. *Nature* 405(6 783): 105-6.

———. 2006. 'South Africa Takes Steps to Tackle HIV'. *Nature* 444(7120): 663.

Colvin, C.J. 2003. 'Contingency and Creativity: South Africa after Apartheid'. *Anthropology and Humanism* 28(1): 3-7.

Das, P. 2005. 'Is Abstinence-Only Threatening Uganda's HIV Success Story?' *Lancet* 5(5): 263-4.

Deane, N. 2005. 'The Political History of AIDS Treatment'. In S.S. Abdool Karim and Q. Abdool Karim (eds). *HIV/AIDS in South Africa*. Cambridge: Cambridge University Press: 538-47.

Dorrington, R., D. Bradshaw and D. Budlender. 2002. *HIV/AIDS Profile in the Provinces of South Africa: Indicators for 2002*. Cape Town: Centre for Actuarial Research, Medical Research Council and the Actuarial Society of South Africa.

'The Durban Declaration'. 2000. *Nature* 406(6 791): 15–16.

Dwyer, P. 2003. 'South Africa: Dying to Fight'. *Review of African Political Economy* 30(98): 661–3.

Geffen, N. 2009. 'Justice after AIDS Denialism: Should There be Prosecutions and Compensation?' *Journal of Acquired Immune Deficiency Syndromes* 51(4): 454–5.

Kunda, L.J. 2006. ' "We Don't Do Plastics": A Critique of the Health Belief Model'. Paper presented at the South African Communication Association, Stellenbosch, 15–16 September.

Liebenberg, I. 1998. 'The African Renaissance: Myth, Vital Lie, or Mobilising Tool?' *African Security Review* 7(3): 42–50.

loveLife. 2001. *Impending Catastrophe Revisited: An Update on the HIV/AIDS Epidemic in South Africa*. Johannesburg: Henry J. Kaiser Family Foundation.

Madlala-Routledge, N. 2006. 'Statement by the Deputy Minister of Health on Media Reports Calling the President to do an AIDS Test'. Available at www.doh.gov.za/show.php?id=1610.

Makgoba, M.W. (ed.). 1999. *African Renaissance: The New Struggle*. Johannesburg: Mafube.

Makgoba, M.W. 2000. 'HIV/AIDS: The Peril of Pseudoscience'. *Science* 288(5 469): 1171.

Marais, H. 2005. *Buckling: The Impact of AIDS in South Africa*. Pretoria: Centre for the Study of Aids.

'Mbeki's Mistake'. 2007. *Nature* 448(7155): 727.

Mbigi, L. 1995. *Ubuntu: The Spirit of African Transformation Management*. Pretoria: Knowledge Resources.

Mbiti, J.S. 1969. *African Religions & Philosophy*. New York: Praeger.

———. 1990. *African Religions & Philosophy* (2nd rev. and enl. ed.). Oxford: Heinemann.

McClelland, S.I. and M. Fine. 2008. 'Embedded Science: Critical Analysis of Abstinence-Only Evaluation Research'. *Cultural Studies, Critical Methodologies* 8(1): 50–81.

Milio, N. 2005. 'Ideology, Science, and Public Policy'. *Journal of Epidemiology and Community Health* 59(10): 814–15.

Moemeka, A.A. 1998. 'Communalism as a Fundamental Dimension of Culture'. *Journal of Communication* 48: 118–41.

Nattrass, N. 2006. *AIDS, Science and Governance: The Battle over Antiretroviral Therapy in Post-Apartheid South Africa*. Cape Town: University of Cape Town.

———. 2007. 'AIDS: Denialism vs. Science'. *Skeptical Inquirer* 31(5): 31–7.

———. 2008. 'Aids and the Scientific Governance of Medicine in Post-Apartheid South Africa'. *African Affairs* 107(427): 157–76.

'News in Brief'. 2007. *Nature* 448(7 155): 739.

Niehaus, I. and G. Jonsson. 2005. 'Dr. Wouter Basson, Americans, and Wild Beasts: Men's Conspiracy Theories of HIV/AIDS in the South African Lowveld' *Medical Anthropology* 24: 179–208.

Nyamiti, C. 1989. *Jesus in African Christianity: Experimentation and Diversity in African Christology.* Nairobi: Initiatives.

Nyonator, F.K., J.K. Awoonor-Williams, J.F. Phillips, T.C. Jones and R.A. Miller. 2005. 'The Ghana Community-Based Health Planning and Services Initiative for Scaling up Service Delivery Innovation'. *Health Policy Plan* 20(1): 25–34.

Oakley, A., V. Strange, C. Bonell, E. Allen, J. Stephenson and R.S. Team. 2006. 'Process Evaluation in Randomised Controlled Trials of Complex Interventions'. *British Medical Journal* 332(7 538): 413–16.

Schneider, H. and D. Fassin. 2002. 'Denial and Defiance: A Socio-Political Analysis of AIDS in South Africa'. *AIDS* 16(4): S45–S51.

Sidley, P. 2006. 'South Africa Sidelines its Health Minister on AIDS Issues'. *British Medical Journal* 333(7 572): 774.

'South Africa's AIDS Plan'. 2007. *Nature* 447(7 140): 1.

South African Press Association. 2008. 'Manto: No Western Trials for Traditional Medicine'. *Mail & Guardian*, 28 February. Available at www.mg.co.za/articlePage.aspx?articleid=333154&area=/breaking_news/breaking_news__national/.

Stoneburner, R.L. and D. Low-Beer. 2004. 'Population-Level HIV Declines and Behavioral Risk Avoidance in Uganda'. *Science* 304(5671): 714–18.

Tempels, P. 1959. *Bantu Philosophy.* Paris: Presence Africaine.

Tomaselli, K. 1999. 'Cultural Studies in Africa: Positioning Difference'. *Critical Arts* 13(1): 1–14.

Tucker, T.J. and M.W. Makgoba. 2008. 'Public Health: Public-Private Partnerships and Scientific Imperialism'. *Science* 320(5 879): 1016–17.

Watson, J. 2005. 'Vitamin Guru Provokes Wrath of Scientists, Activists'. *Nature Medicine* 11: 581.

Wendo, C. 2003. 'Bush's Visit to Uganda Raises Hopes and Sparks Controversy'. *Lancet* 362(9 379): 216–17.

Younde, J. 2007. 'Ideology's Role in AIDS Policies in Uganda and South Africa'. *Global Health Governance* 1(1): 1–16.

Zeleza, P.T. (ed.). 2006. *Selected Proceedings of the 36th Annual Conference on African Linguistics.* Somerville, MA: Cascadilla Proceedings Project.

6

President Jammeh's HIV/AIDS Healing Saga in The Gambia

Stella Nyanzi

With a population of less than two million people, The Gambia is the smallest country in West Africa. The first incidence of HIV was diagnosed in 1986. Initial state response to HIV/AIDS was slow, shrouded by secrecy and denial. However, external donor funding facilitated public health interventions aimed at prevention, treatment and care, as well as community-based support. There is limited access to free antiretroviral (ARV) therapies in specific centres. According to UNAIDS (2007), HIV prevalence in the general population of adults aged 15–49 years is 2.4% and is mainly transmitted through unprotected heterosexual contact. Among women attending antenatal clinics, prevalence of HIV-1 is 1.0% and HIV-2 is 0.8% (Van der Loeff et al. 2003).

The Gambia's president, Yahya Jammeh, publicly announced his HIV/AIDS cure in January 2007. He announced that he was a *marabout* (healer/guide) who possessed the cure for HIV/AIDS, which was revealed to him by Allah in a dream. Using his influence and powerful position, he recruited 'batches' of people infected with HIV to the state house, insisted that they abandon ARV therapy and administered his regimen.[1]

This chapter explores the interplay between the authority of the state, of science and the local psyche of Islamic healing. It unpacks the layers of conflicts and compromises that occurred through President Yahya Jammeh. The chapter is based on ethnographic fieldwork conducted between 2002 and 2008, but here I focus on the events surrounding the president's programme during 2007 and 2008 and draw largely on statements by the president to examine the rhetoric used to promote his cure programme and the public performances of power. The critical question at the heart of this chapter, following Nyanzi and Bah (2008), is: 'Who protects the subjects when Science and the State collude to promote a counterfeit cure'?

During a meeting in the Cabinet room on 18 January 2007, President Yahya Jammeh announced that he was starting public treatment of HIV/AIDS and asthma. Dignitaries present that afternoon included the management of the Royal Victoria Teaching Hospital (RVTH), several secretaries of state, the ambassadors of Cuba and Taiwan, and Rose Claire Charles, a United Nations' volunteer working with the Santa Yalla Support Society (SYSS) for HIV-infected people. The president presented his intention as a directive from powers beyond himself and revealed that he had previously provided successful private non-biomedical therapies for diverse conditions to many people and it was now time for him to offer a public service:

> I call you to this meeting and maybe you will wonder why I called you including the two Ambassadors from Cuba and Taiwan. I called in the two Ambassadors and of course Rose Claire Charles because you have a direct link with the health delivery system of this country. You know that Cuba is a key partner in our health sector and Taiwan is the force behind the Medical Team in The Gambia. This is a follow up to what I said on GRTS [Gambian Radio and Television Services] that I will now fully participate in the treatment of certain critical cases.
>
> Since 1994, there are many Gambians who know what I can do. A lot of people have been treated in silence or under

conditions of strict confidentiality. One would wonder why I start giving medicine to the public and all of a sudden stop. I have been having a lot of queries about that even after we went to the RVTH on Saturday. People were saying, 'Well, the President. This is what he does. He will introduce very effective medicines and all of a sudden it will die down and we will not have access to him.'

I had to work on instructions. I don't have the mandate to do it publicly in great numbers. I was only restricted to a small number so as to be able to prove to people that what I say is what I can do before I have the permission to do it publicly.

I am not speculating on my medicine. There are living witnesses to what my medicine can do. As far as I am concerned it takes only five minutes to cure asthma. I have other medicinal herbs that can take care of a number of illnesses. One of it was the one that was sold publicly at the July 22 Square and the Serrekunda Police Station. But of course, it has to stop at a point because I don't have the mandate to go beyond that. I now have the mandate to cure people publicly under strict conditions that I have to abide by otherwise I pay the price.

Now I have the mandate to publicly treat all the diseases on condition that the patient will be treated publicly. In fact, the first and the most important condition is that the person must be diagnosed by a medical practitioner or a medical institution. I am not authorised to treat anybody who just feels sick without a doctor's confirmation. I can treat asthma and HIV/AIDS and the cure is a day's treatment. Within three days that person should be tested again and I can tell you that he/she will be negative. After the treatment, they have to go to the RVTH for a test again. As I said, I will not treat anybody who is not diagnosed as asthmatic or a HIV/AIDS patient by a doctor. I don't want to give my medicine to a wrong person. So the reason why I called you is that I have to work with a team of doctors that I can trust. Doctors who will not sabotage my treatment. That does not in any way mean that I will give them the medicine. Those doctors would make sure that the patients abide by the instructions. If I give you the medicine with instructions on how to go about it and you go and do something contrary to that and you turn out to be positive, don't blame me. I will not give you names but it is true. It is not a treatment that I speculate on. I am not doing it for money or popularity. The mandate I have is that HIV/AIDS can be treated on Thursdays. That is the good news and the bad news is that I cannot treat more than ten patients every Thursday. There is nothing I can do about it and if I go beyond that I will have to pay the price.

For asthma, I have to choose between Saturday and Friday. I am also not authorised to treat more than 100 people. I am also not authorised to treat anybody who does not produce a diagnostic paper or asthma or HIV/AIDS. One will asked what the Cuban and Taiwanese ambassadors are doing here. The aim is to share the treatment with them because in Taiwan traditional medicines are used. The asthma medicine can be mass produced and packaged and exported to them. The one on HIV/AIDS cannot be mass produced because I am restricted to ten patients only on every Thursday and I cannot go beyond that. I want to have a team of three doctors for asthma and HIV/AIDS. I want you to select ten HIV/AIDS patients: five males and five females for Thursday.

The conditions should be explained to them before they come because if any of them backs out, you cannot replace the one that has backed out. They can eat before coming but they should not eat anything that is oily. The medicine will be given to them in the morning as a preliminary and after, they can eat and in the evening they take it again. Once that is done, they cannot eat anything else the following morning. They may be hungry and thirsty but they have to bear it and that is why they need a doctor to monitor them. Once they have taken the medicine, they should not eat anything no matter what happens till the following day.

Now with regards to asthma treatment, that is the easiest part. When they are coming for treatment in the morning, they should not eat anything that has pepper or seafood when they take the medicine, for four hours they should not eat anything. After that they can eat anything except something that contains oil or seafood. We want to see how we can work with the RVTH to see where these people can be kept until the following morning. With regards to asthma treatment, there is no need to keep them. They can go for six months, without taking anything that is alcoholic. With regards to HIV/AIDS, they should be kept at a place that has adequate toilet facilities because they can be going to toilet every five minutes. Anybody who says he will not be treated publicly should stay away because I have to fulfil the conditions and will not take risks for anybody.

I am not a witch doctor and in fact you cannot have a witch doctor. You are either a witch or a doctor.[2]

The presidential statement attests to a turning point in the trajectory of HIV/AIDS discourse, policy and practice in The Gambia. Establishing a characteristic pattern, the president later granted interviews to representatives of local, regional and international media houses.

The president's HIV/AIDS cure programme

A group of nine HIV-infected Gambians was recruited after screening and admitted to the 'Glass House' (the president's treatment centre) in the state house, where they were subjected to a strict regimen. The admission criteria initially included: Gambian nationality, proven medical diagnosis of HIV infection and agreement to allow the treatment to be publicised. Later batches were subjected to diagnosis through full medical history, physical examinations and laboratory investigation (including voluntary counselling and testing at Serrekunda Hospital), blood tests (including viral loads and CD4 counts), urine tests and chest X-rays. Some facts outlining the programme are:

- The first batch of 9 people was admitted on 18 January 2007, comprising only Gambian adults;

- The second batch of 27 people, including 3 infants, was admitted on 14 February 2007;
- The third batch of 38 people was admitted on 17 April 2007;
- The fourth batch of 32 people, including 7 foreigners from Guinea, Senegal, Malawi and Ivory Coast was admitted on 9 August 2007.

On 31 July 2007, the first and second batches of people living with HIV/AIDS (PLWHA) were discharged, with pronouncements that they were cured. By mid-2008, four batches of HIV-infected patients had received the presidential HIV/AIDS cure.

Proclaiming that he had instructions from a higher being, the president declared that the effectiveness of his treatment was conditional upon total adherence to a list of prohibitions that included no sexual intercourse (even between spouses), no alcohol, cigarettes, coffee, Chinese green tea or any biomedical pharmaceuticals. It was also mandatory for his admitted patients to cease ARV therapies. In all related speeches, the president repeatedly issued stern warnings against the use of scientific, 'Western' or biomedical medicines throughout the treatment period. Additionally, his patients were required to meet special food observances, including a strict schedule of eating and refraining from eating, as well as prohibitions against ingesting anything provided from outside his premises. The latter prerequisite was based on suspicions of malicious factions with potential to contaminate or otherwise poison patients' food and thereby discredit the president's cure. Strict adherence to these conditions was a measure of the patients' commitment to the president's healing programme. Failure to comply led to immediate expulsion as was publicised in the following statement:

> It is also important to tell Gambians that we have cause to expel three patients who violated all our rules, which was detrimental to the well-being of the patients. One from the first group, two from the second group. In the third group, as far as I know, we have no cause to expel anybody, but the rules are very clear. Violate the rules, repeat it and go home. I will not take risk.[3]

Claiming his sole motivation was a deep desire to restore the well-being of his Gambian subjects, Jammeh administered a combination of herbal concoctions, presidential massage, Islamic prayer, chanting and counselling. Despite the label 'herbal treatment' the therapeutic regimen included syncretism of several non-biomedical therapies. He explained that the cure composed of 10% herbs and 90% 'the Almighty Allah'. He also asserted he was driven by neither popularity nor profit but by the redemption of humanity, particularly 'Black Africans' and the benevolence of God:

> Why today? I don't claim to be God, I don't claim to be a prophet but I've every right to claim that am a God fearing person and my love for humanity have no limit and I do everything possible to please the Almighty Allah, and I prayed to Allah. Am not looking for popularity, wealth, but all what I seek is the pleasure of the Almighty Allah. We are not visitors of this world, we are leaving today. The most important world that we all aspire of is the Kingdom of Allah in heaven. Whatever I do in this world, I do in pursuit of the next world.[4]

However, he conducted several press interviews and consistently issued press releases, including to the international media. New developments in the programme were updated on the Gambian state house web pages and regularly broadcast via GRTS. Furthermore, an account was opened at the Arab Gambia Islamic Bank to receive financial support for the presidential HIV/AIDS treatment programme. A press release issued by the Department of State for Health and Social Welfare, states:

> The above mentioned Department is hereby informing the general public that the Trust Fund in the treatment of HIV/AIDS and other diseases by His Excellency The President is lodged with the AGIB bank.
> The name of the fund is 'Dr Yahya AJJ Jammeh Trust Fund for the treatment of HIV/AIDS and other diseases' Account Number 21160120380019.

All individuals, groups, companies and organisations, who wish to donate towards the fund could do so at the AGIB Bank.[5]

Yahya Jammeh: The healer

Nor does it surprise me that people are lining up, begging to be treated by the president. Faith healers abound. *Marabouts*, a combination of priest, sage, mystic, prophet and healer, with their specially prepared *jujus* (amulets), sometimes containing bits of wild animals and Qur'anic verses often written with a bone from a black cat in blood from the same cat, are consulted on a daily basis. The *marabouts* appear to be the holders and guardians of truth. I have rarely met someone who did not believe in the power of the *marabout* or in the power of *jujus*. *Marabouts* are not questioned: they are assumed to be experts, and their truth is THE truth. They are the scholars, teachers, healers and diviners. In ancient times they were the judges in the councils of the kings. In fact, one man tells me that the '*marabout* is The Gambian scientist'. And another man tells me that 'Jammeh is the best, the most powerful, *marabout*' (Starin 2007a: 295).

Considering the epithets that have been coined about Yahya Jammeh (for example, 'medical myth buster', 'doctor among doctors' and 'Africa's messiah'), he seemed to have won himself credibility as a healer in The Gambian's public discourse. But who is Yahya Jammeh?

Born on 25 May 1965 in Kanilai village, in Foni Kansala District in the Western Division, he adopted the names Yahya Abdul Azziz Jemus Junkung Jammeh. Divorced from a Gambian Muslim (Darboe 2004: 79), he married Zineb Jammeh, of Moroccan descent, and they have two children. He attended St Anthony's School (1972-6), St Edward's Primary School, Bwiam (1976-8) and passed common entrance examinations in 1978. On government scholarship at Gambia High School (1978-83), he obtained credits in Geography, English, French, Biology and Physics, and passes in Chemistry and Oral English in the General Certificate of Education examinations.

He joined Gambia National Gendarmerie's Special Intervention Unit in 1984. In 1986 he was promoted from private to sergeant and served in the Mobile Gendarmerie and Special Guards Unit. In 1987 he was promoted to cadet officer and joined the Gendarmerie Training School, specifically the School of Presidential Escort. In 1989 he was commissioned. Between 1991 and 1994, he was officer commanding of the Mobile Gendarmerie, the Military Police Unit of the Gambia National Gendarmerie and the Gambia National Army at Yumdum Barracks. Promotion to ranks of second lieutenant, lieutenant, captain and colonel came in 1989, 1992, 1994 and 1996 respectively. On 22 July 1994, this 'chronically destitute' youngster who had reportedly enlisted in the army to 'escape unemployment and permanent lumpenisation' (Kandeh 1996: 391) overthrew the regime in a bloodless *coup d'état*, to become head of state and chairman of the Armed Forces Provisional Ruling Council (Loum 2002; Saine 1996; Wiseman and Vidler 1995; Wiseman 1996). Under international pressure for democratic elections, he formed a new political party and conducted presidential elections. He retired from the army on 8 September 1996. On 27 September of the same year, he was elected first president of the Second Republic of The Gambia.

His grip on the presidency has carried through three elections, despite being contested by the opposition and academic scholars (Edie 2000; Wiseman 1997; Saine 2008a, 2008b, 2000a, 1997). The regime reportedly violated diverse principles of democracy. The 1996 presidential election was disputed due to multiple irregularities, including vote-buying, illegitimate voter registration, rigging, flawed appeal structure dependent on the incumbent, doctoring the Constitution, intimidation and violence against the opposition, illicit votes from non-Gambian members of Jammeh's Jola ethnic group who crossed over from the Cassamance and an electoral commission chairman who manipulated the rules (Edie 2000: 169, 170; Saine 2002b: 168). Democratisation processes in this era were described as a 'moldy loaf' (Wiseman 1998). Developing this metaphor, Saine (2002a: 171) likened the subsequent 2001 elections to a 'moldier loaf' (see also Edie 2000: 185, 193; Schweisfurth 2002 for discussion about local interpretations of democracy). All these flaws, including repression of the press, opposition parties and dissidents, were heightened in the 2006 presidential elections (Saine 2008a). In addition to widespread voter intimidation by local chiefs, governors and security guards, the president 'threatened to single out for punishment those who did not vote for him by depriving their constituency of aid' (Saine 2008a: 167).

Regarding the source of his power, the president explained he had inherited special healing abilities from his father who belonged to a lineage of traditional herbalists, Islamic healers and spiritual healers. He further claimed that the cure for HIV/AIDS was revealed to him in a dream. Notably, Jammeh is of Jola ethnicity and his culture is renowned for a highly developed system of alternative medicine combining herbs (*jujus*), spirits (*sinaati*), fertility cults, Islamic scriptures, holy water (*naaso*), spirit shrines (*enarte*) and sacred groves, which are provided by many practitioners including herbalists (*amori*), hunters (*ahweema*), herdsmen (*ah-hawa*), midwives (*ahjogar gukonya nganogen*) and healers (*marabouts*) (Madge 1998).

Jammeh has sometimes alluded to divine appointment, as justification for his power. For example, he has claimed that his name and instructions are in the Qur'an. He has been depicted as 'a devout Muslim with an abiding sense of mission and empathy for the poor' (Kandeh 1996: 395) but critics such as Wiseman decipher this image as:

> the calculatingly invented public image of the military leader which [Jammeh] is anxious to project for political reasons. Around six months after the coup, pin-up pictures of Jammeh dressed in battle fatigues which had been widely available on the streets of Banjul, were replaced by new ones depicting him as a holy man at prayer (1997: 266).

Saine further elaborates:

> Jammeh's ostentatious adoption of a Muslim public image was as much to do with building up domestic and external support as with personal belief . . . motivated primarily by his desire to

attract a lot of foreign assistance, including funds for development projects as well as the construction of mosques around
the country (2000b: 80).

Finally, Darboe's description rounds up the literature about Jammeh's
relationship to Islam: 'President Yahya Jammeh, a master of
manipulation of Islamic symbols . . . has frequently blurred the line
between mosque and state to reinforce his political advantage . . .
illustrates the reciprocal relationship between religion and politics and
politicians' use of Islam for personal gain' (2004: 73).

The creative (mis)appropriation of biomedical science
Biomedicine and African indigenous medicinal systems are distinct
therapeutic paradigms but there is overlap (Last and Chavunduka 1986;
Van der Geest 1997). Characteristically, each has its own well-developed
procedures of illness classification, diagnosis, prognosis, prescription
and treatment. However, Yahya Jammeh espoused a convergence by
insisting that it was mandatory for individuals to produce evidence of
clinical diagnosis of HIV based on laboratory tests prior to enrolling
for his cure. He justified this requirement by insisting it was central to
his mystical mandate, to verify he was actually curing HIV/AIDS and
not other ailments, and it would be a basis for confirming his cure if
the virus was no longer found in the body upon completion of the
treatment.

From a biomedical perspective, most viruses are self-eliminating
microbes without cures per se. HIV has no biomedical cure yet. Once
inside the body, it replicates rapidly and also continuously mutates.
ARV therapies counter its replication. Claiming to totally 'cure' HIV-
infected people within three, ten or fifteen days, the president revealed
a lack of understanding of HIV as a complex virological entity and
went beyond the approach of alternative therapies. Alternative medical
therapies mostly lay claims to 'healing', as opposed to 'curing', which
is very specific to biomedical conceptions of disease (Feierman and
Janzen 1992), but the president proclaimed a convergence of the two
therapeutic paradigms.

There was overt use of biomedical language in press releases about his treatment. For instance, the initial release of laboratory test results of the HIV-infected people enrolled in the president's programme included references to different levels of 'viral load', 'virus undetectable' and 'screening batches'. Evidence of a 'successful cure' was given in tabular illustrations showing results with numerical values for copies of virus per millilitre of blood. Distinctions of results for HIV-1 and HIV-2 were often provided.

The technical jargon provided a veneer of high-sounding sophistication, particularly for Gambian audiences, but it was not scientifically credible. For example, reference to a reduction in viral load to undetectable limits does not mean total elimination of the virus; it speaks to the power of detection of laboratory test mechanisms and omits the fact that polymerase chain reaction (PCR) tests cannot detect the virus in some parts of the body, such as the brain. Nonetheless, the reports revealed both the complicity of biomedical technocrats and the directing of the communication to Gambians and to external agencies. Excerpts of statements from the state house below clearly illustrate this point:

> Well for the rest of the people that have not been discharged, I made it very clear that it is my responsibility and I have explained clearly what my medicine does to HIV/AIDS. What I said, I will repeat it. I will get rid of the AIDS virus in your bodies. Those who we think the virus is finished in their body, are those discharged. I made it clear. But if you even have 10 copies in your body, I will not let you go until these 10 copies are eliminated from your body.[6]

There is ample evidence based on western scientific verification methods, through laboratory tests conducted by medical professors at the faculty of medicine, Cheikh Anta Diop University, Dakar, Senegal, that patients who were tested HIV positive prior to commencement of treatment were again tested after the treatment and the results showed that the virus became undetectable. That is to say the virus can no longer be seen, which in layman's language and to the patients affected, the disease had been conquered. What other proofs are people still asking for? President Jammeh does not have to convince anyone that he has been given the gift and knowledge to cure AIDS. And he does not have to explain to anyone the secrets of this gift and knowledge to cure AIDS.[7]

Confidentiality is critical to the biomedical care and treatment of HIV/ AIDS, particularly on the part of healthcare providers, with the prerogative left to HIV-infected individuals to decide whether to disclose their status and to whom. However, participation in the president's programme revoked this principle. Individuals' names, pictures, films, repeated HIV-test details, narratives of experiences and interviews were broadcast through diverse media. Ironically, an unintended and positive effect was to lift the veil of denial about AIDS in The Gambia (Shaw and Jawo 2000; Nyanzi 2009).

The precondition to abandon ARV treatment was a serious breach of HIV-infected people's commitment to adherence to their biomedical therapy. There were appeals to reveal the contents of his 'cure', particularly his herbal concoctions, to the scientific community so that they could conduct tests on safety, efficacy, dosage, potential side effects, pharmacological ingredients and chemical actions. However, these requests were refused; the ingredients are secret to the president's family and the knowledge held by only 'specially chosen individuals' (Madge 1998: 302).

This secrecy is a typical characteristic of indigenous therapies (Van der Geest 1997). Furthermore, issues such as dosage and efficacy are Western biomedical constructs, not necessarily relevant in many herbal remedies (Helman 2002). This point highlights the inherent clash of therapeutic paradigms in their criteria of evaluation. The requirements essential to meeting the standards of good therapy in biomedical science contrast sharply with the tenets of indigenous medicine.

The Gambian president resisted scientific debate about his cure but also proclaimed scientific merit for his programme, often in extraordinarily bombastic ways. For example on an Al Jazeera broadcast, he disparaged a leading African scientist, Professor Jerry Hoosain Coovadia, who disclaimed the plausibility of the HIV/AIDS cure. Quelling any debate, Jammeh retorted:

> He doesn't know anything about AIDS. Maybe he is among those who made the virus . . . I don't owe that idiot any explanation because he is an idiot. Who is he to talk about what I do? He doesn't know anything about science . . . We shouldn't waste time talking about such a fool.

In one instance, in relation to an appointment for a new secretary of state for higher education, research, science and technology, he asserted: 'We cannot continue to depend on other country's scientists for our national development requirements. You will train people who will be conducting research for our country's requirements'.[8]

In another instance, a state house statement described results of analyses reportedly conducted by Professor Rajae El Aouad, the director of the Moroccan National Institute of Hygiene, as 'proof that ten out of the forty HIV patients have no virus in their blood'.[9] Another tactic was to issue press releases, which included name-dropping to infer scientific credibility and institutional backing; for instance, citing the use of tests also used by renowned Senegalese clinicians (who had worked to discover the HIV-2 virus), Professors Coumba Toure Kane and Soulayman Mboup at Cheikh Anta Diop University. The professors replied through the International AIDS Society and Society for AIDS in Africa (IAS and SAA 2007), distancing themselves from the president's claims and emphasising that no conclusion about the treatment could be made because of the absence of evidence on the use of necessary scientific measures (for example, baseline data and different data points).

At the end of March 2008, a statement on laboratory tests for 21 patients presented an impression of scientific rigour but it was deceptive.[10] For example, after name entries there was a column entitled 'PCR result for HIV 1 (IU/ml) 17/10/2007', with individuals' results ranging from 74 to 63 625 126. Adjacent was another column entitled

'PCR result for HIV 1 (IU/ml) 18/3/2008' with four entries of 'below detection limit' and the rest with numeric values much less than corresponding entries in the preceding column. The last column was entitled 'PCR result for HIV 2 (Copies/ml) 18/3/2008)', with five entries of 'undetected', one with the number 529 and the rest with a dash. This presentation inferred a drop in the viral load of patients with HIV-1 within a period of five months and, if a reader did not check that the last column referred to HIV-2, a suggestion of elimination of the virus. There were other inconsistencies. For example, the use of different measurements, 'International Units' and 'Copies' (per millilitre) is confusing and inappropriate. There is also no basis to attribute the decrease in viral load to a specific cause because of gaps in evidence presented. Notably, there was no clear indication of the gap in time between when patients stopped taking ARVs and started taking the presidential cure; hence, whether or not there were continued effects of ARVs.

A key feature of the president's cure programme was the co-option of health professionals in The Gambia. From the outset, the secretary of state for health and social welfare, Dr Tamsir Mbowe, supported the president. Mbowe is a physician, trained in Ukraine and Ireland. Pictures place him with the president, participating in the screening, recruitment, treatment and counselling of HIV-infected patients and, alongside the president's speeches when admitting and discharging the different batches of HIV-infected people, there was a list of Mbowe's speeches. Appended to all early press releases about the cure, there was the following statement: 'For any information on the President's on-going treatment of HIV infection, please contact Dr. Tamsir Mbowe, Secretary of State for Health and Social Welfare on 9914535/ 7764535'. The following press release is a good example of both the president's use of scientific language, as discussed above, as well as Dr Mbowe's collusion:

> Reports of the first test results of the nine HIV infected persons being treated by the President Yahya Jammeh have revealed that the CD4 count (special T-lymphocyte) of the patients have gone

up 'impressively', signifying a marked improvement on the patients from a laboratory point of view.

According to the revelation, seven out of the nine patients have their CD4 counts ranging from 200 to over 1300 as compared to when they first reported for treatment, barely ten days ago, recording CD4 counts of less than 50.

The HIV/AIDS treatment began January 18, 2007, following President Jammeh's disclosure of a 'mandate' to cure HIV/AIDS and asthma patients. The patients were treated on the conditions that they are diagnosed by a medical practitioner and that they are treated publicly.

Speaking to GRTS, after the release of the test result, President Jammeh expressed confidence that any person with HIV/AIDS who comes to his clinic will not die. President Jammeh asserted that the duration of the treatment ranges from three to ten days and or from twenty to thirty days.

President Jammeh said he was pleased to note that the nine patients who were very low on their CD4 count, have made considerable improvement. According to President Jammeh, when the patients first arrived at the glass house for treatment, some of them could hardly stand on their feet for 2 minutes. He noted the remarkable improvement within ten days of treatment of a particular patient who had been infected for 2 years and nine months, with the highest score on CD4 count. 'We had a problem with him because we had to force him before he takes the medicine. Even to apply on his body was a big problem,' President Jammeh stated.

The Gambian leader further added that he will make sure that all the patients regain their health since most of them had very big problems with their internal organs like the intestines. 'The women, in particular, had chronic problems,' he added. The President then revealed that as of now, all the patients are cough-free, among other things. 'They can even run if I want them to run. So they are very OK now,' he assured.

For his part, Dr Tamsir Mbowe, Secretary of State for Health and Social Welfare explained that the results are really very impressive and excellent. He said most of the patients, presently have a CD 4 count of between 195 to 1338.

This, according to him, is excellent news and means that the treatment is going very fine and there is marked improvement in the patients' condition from a laboratory point of view. 'In order to be on ARV's, you must have your CD 4 count at 200 or below. Now out of the 9 patients President Jammeh is treating, 7 have their CD4 counts above 200, while one have 450, 500, 750, 834 to 1334,' he said.

Dr Mbowe then stated that: 'This clearly shows that the treatment is very effective and we are really having gains now, which can be declared to the whole world. Before the treatment, we had patients who had a CD 4 count of less than 50 and are now having increment in their CD4 level from about 200 to 1334. I am very much comfortable and happy with the treatment,' he explained.[11]

Many people in The Gambia questioned Dr Mbowe's professional ethics; a common explanation being that he succumbed to the 'politics of the belly'. This was a reference to the nature of ministerial politics in the country: 'Jammeh dismisses his ministers when they no longer serve his political ends. He has also been known to use them as scapegoats when problems arise that he has no solutions to' (Saine 2000b: 83). According to Wiseman, 'when indulging in the frequent exercise of sacking ministers Jammeh routinely accuses them of large-scale corruption' (1997: 266).

Dr Mbowe later relinquished his position as secretary of state and became the director-general of the Presidential Medical Team.[12] Malick Njie was appointed the subsequent secretary of state for health and Sulayman Samba as permanent secretary for health. During celebrations of the first anniversary of the presidential AIDS cure, both Njie and Samba were recorded as 'pledging unflinching support to the presidential HIV/AIDS cure'.[13]

In addition, the president embellished his claims of scientific credibility with images of medical personnel involved in the programme. Early media releases highlight Cuban medical interns working alongside the president and Dr Mbowe, as they administered the HIV/AIDS 'cure'.[14] Pictorial evidence confirms their involvement in the therapeutic rituals of the first batch. However, their involvement was short-lived, for reasons that are not clear. The public was informed:

> Well, to our Cuban brothers and sisters, these are true friends of The Gambia. Today Gambia's profile in the medical service is among the best in the whole world. Thanks to the generosity of the Cuban government and people. Well they may be wondering why, they don't continue on the treatment. When we started, we started with them. Then a situation arose and I have to let them go. The reason being, when the first CD4 counts results were announced I realised that we have picked a huge fight globally and since the valiant people of Cuba has always been in fight in big powers. I don't want them to be part of another global fight. I pick up the fight on behalf of The Gambia and humanity. I didn't want to add another burden to the republic of Cuba, that was the only reason why I said we leave our Cuban brothers and sisters in peace, while we continue this global fight that has been unleashed on us. So, it is not because you are not efficient it is not that we did not trust you, the simple reason is that I don't want to put you in a fight that is directly against Yahya Jammeh and The Gambia. The principles of humanity dictates us that, if you have a friend who is always in a fight and trying to help you, it's more honourable to involve him in a new fight. That is the reason why our Cuban sisters and brothers were relieved of their responsibility in the treatment of HIV/AIDS.[15]

In summary, the president has been a master manipulator and strategist. He has used medical professionals to lend credibility to his programme and thereby sustain public interest in it and, in particular, ensure a constant flow of HIV-infected people seeking to be cured. As I have intimated, Jammeh's rhetoric was infused with political inferences. I will discuss this aspect of his agenda in more detail below.

The politics of HIV/AIDS in The Gambia

President Jammeh's discourse on HIV/AIDS aptly expresses Amon's argument: 'ART [antiretroviral therapy] programs inevitably exist in the political sphere and, as we have seen, governments use the promotion of unproven AIDS remedies as part of larger political campaigns to express benevolence or promote "indigenous" solutions' (2008: 7).

In 2007, the president expelled a United Nations official who questioned the credibility and potential negative consequences of his HIV/AIDS programme (Reuters 2007; Amon 2008: 3). Subsequently, the United Nations, the Joint United Nations Programme on HIV/AIDS (UNAIDS) and the World Health Organization (WHO) published statements emphasising that there was still no cure for AIDS and that replacing scientifically researched treatments with untested therapies could lead to adverse effects including death (United Nations 2007; UNAIDS and WHO 2007; WHO 2007). In response, President Jammeh lambasted these organisations:

> I will never waver my crusade in the fight against HIV in The Gambia and in Africa. Yes you will be surprised to know that the WHO and the UNAIDS have given endless problems to the laboratories that tested the blood samples and proven that the medicine is effective. Now they want to know where we want to go next so that they can go and talk to that country not to accept samples from The Gambia. Why? There is a reason. Even we Gambians believe in witchcraft. When somebody dies and it is claimed that the person may be killed by witchcrafts, even thought those who are suspected of killing the person cry the most. Yes, because they don't want to show that they are responsible for the person's death. So those who produce AIDS to kill Africans (blacks) are the ones crying loud about doing

something about AIDS in Africa. But their insincerity has been shown by their brutal attacks on something that scientifically cannot be disputed, that is the results of my treatment. If they are concerned about HIV/AIDS and they want to stop it, if they are sincere, the first thing they should have done was to come and say let's see how we can develop it and make it available for humanity . . .

Now, everybody believes the statistics the western press gives about Africa. They have shown all laboratory evidence to back their claim that in some countries, 3 out of 4 nationals are HIV positive. The UNAIDS and WHO accepted those figures. So, why can't the UNAIDS and WHO accepted laboratory test that are more evident proven than what these people are claiming because our resources is tested in a modern laboratory for that matter. So if they are concerned about the AIDS pandemic in Africa, why can't they embrace any attempt that shows positive signs that AIDS can be taken care of?[16]

In the same speech, the president overtly projected himself as a representative of oppressed 'black' Africa championing a struggle against a 'Western' conspiracy to kill Africans:

The fight against HIV/AIDS, the treatment has exposed the hypocrisy and lip service that the western world is putting on today. Let us ask ourselves as African and Non-Europeans, why is AIDS killing more blacks and than the rest of humanity? . . .

By the grace of Allah, we will continue to treat AIDS, asthma and diabetes.

Less overt was the propagation of a particular Islamic discourse that emphasises cultural difference and division between 'the West' and Islam.[17] Nonetheless, as is evident from the preceding discussion, Jammeh's proclamations about his cure are infused with racial and cultural stereotyping to support his claims and to answer his critics.

The president's remarkable rhetoric was, however, only the external expression of his equally remarkable manipulation of presidential and government authority. As Amon has noted: 'The uncertainty and fear engendered by this incurable, stigmatizing and life-threatening disease can make people easy prey to promises of cures. But in addition to fear, there are specific factors, related to government functioning that facilitate false claims of HIV cures' (2008: 1).

The office of the president is mandated to 'uphold and defend the Constitution as the supreme law of The Gambia'. The president is supposed to listen to the voice of the people, represented through Parliament, and act after consultation with the body of technocrats situated within each department of state and linked through a Cabinet minister known as a secretary of state in The Gambia. In addition to Parliament and the ministries, there are other structures such as the judiciary, national assembly, security organs, civil society, public media, research institutions and universities who have various roles to monitor, curb and eliminate the abuse of presidential power.

However in The Gambia, President Jammeh's personal values and unorthodox practices hijacked the systems and processes of accountability and contestation. He employed tactics of alienation, fear, coercion, intimidation, expulsion, exile and oppression to silence any critical voices and thus mute opposition. Surrounding himself with sycophants who only lauded his actions he froze any channels advocating accountability or questioning the credibility, safety, benefit or effectiveness of his HIV/AIDS 'cure'. Notably, people feared the National Intelligence Agency, which the president used to quell dissent and which had reputation for torture, sometimes to the point of death and for destroying property.

As discussed above, several key individuals at the highest levels of decision-making in the Department of State for Health and Social Welfare (notably, Drs Tamsir Mbowe, Mariatou Jallow and Malick Njie) participated in the presidential HIV/AIDS programme, even though they were trained, qualified and experienced physicians. Others such as Dr Pach Njie, chief executive of RVTH and former military physician, lauded the therapy in public.[18]

The RVTH and the Serrekunda Hospital were sites for screening, testing and recruiting patients into the president's programme. The Department of State for Health and Social Welfare endorsed the programme by issuing advertisements, announcing calls for new patient recruitments, broadcasting the schedules and progress reports and providing resources. The National AIDS Secretariat (NAS) was located in the president's office. The NAS is the co-ordination and administration arm of the National AIDS Council (NAC), which is responsible for overseeing the preparation and execution of the national HIV/AIDS strategies and plans for action, as well as implementation of the national 'HIV/AIDS Rapid Response Programme' activities.[19] Reputedly, the SYSS and Nganiye Kiling Society, the two oldest organisations that support and represent PLWHA, were the sources for patients in the president's programme. Rose Claire Charles (a long-time United Nations volunteer working with SYSS) and Lamin Ceesay (the first person in The Gambia to publicly disclose his HIV-positive status) participated in the screening processes for patients.

The reasons for positive press commentary on the programme in The Gambia are not difficult to find. The secretary of state for communications and information technology, Neneh MacDouall-Gaye, was also the chairperson of the Presidential Treatment Support Team. Two journalists lost their jobs at a pro-government newspaper in February 2007 for writing analytical articles about the HIV/AIDS 'cure' (International Freedom of Expression Exchange 2007a, 2007b).

Suppression of press freedom is a known, longstanding feature of politics in The Gambia (Starin 2007b; Saine 2008a; CPJ 2008; Saine 2002b; Hughes 2000). The Media Commission Bill and subsequent amendments to the Criminal Act made 'false publications' punishable by up to one year in prison, or bail set exorbitantly high at 250 000 dalasis (approximately US$9 800). For example, after the government accused *Foroyaa* – an opposition paper of being libellous and in support of treason plots, there ensued a series of court cases, imposition of fines and temporary closures of the newspaper.

Journalists critical of the regime have suffered imprisonment without trial; torture and intimidation; torching of their home compounds, property or vehicles; searches of their office premises; inexplicable disappearances and even mysterious deaths (Reporters without Borders 2008). For instance, Deyda Hydara, the editor of *The Point* newspaper and correspondent for *Agence France* and Reporters without Borders was assassinated on 16 December 2004.[20] Ebrima Manneh, a journalist with the *Observer* newspaper was arrested on 7 July 2006, detained without trial for several months, moved to many police stations and later disappeared, reputedly at the hands of the National Intelligence Agency. Pro-democracy journalist Fatou Jaw Manneh was arrested as she got off an aeroplane to attend her father's funeral, detained at the National Intelligence Agency headquarters in Banjul, accused of sedition, barred from leaving the country and subjected to a long period of trial. Abdoulie Sey, Lamin Fatty, Madi Ceesay and Musa Saidykhan, of *The Independent* newspaper, were jailed and fined large sums of money. The president ordered the arrest and detention of Malick Jones, chief producer of the state-run GRTS, and Mam Sait Ceesay, communications director of the Presidency. Some journalists have fled the country (CPJ 2008).

The local scholarly community has remained silent. There is one university in The Gambia, which was established by the president in 2000. A prominent university lecturer at the School of Public Health was among the first HIV-infected people to receive the HIV/AIDS 'cure'. His story and pictures were revealed in media broadcasts about the programme. Conspicuous for their silence are the academic scientists and researchers based at the Medical Research Council (MRC) Laboratories, the first national referral centre for HIV/AIDS. Some Gambians in the diaspora suspect that speaking out against the president's programme could result in termination of work permits for the numerous foreign staff working in The Gambia. Personal communication with the director of the MRC revealed that he advised his staff members not to get involved in this area on grounds that they: 'have no expertise in Traditional Medicine. This advice is also extended to all students who have links with the Unit in The Gambia and I will advise against you coming to The Gambia to investigate' (18 February 2008).

The absence of strong civil society associations in The Gambia (Edie 2000: 193) contributes to a lack of public debate on the president's programme. Some associations have publicly supported the president. Professional bodies such as the Medical Association or the Bar Association, which have voiced dissent in other matters, have been silent.

Dire repercussions for criticising the presidential HIV/AIDS programme were applied to anyone, regardless of their vocation, rank or nationality. Fadzai Gwaradzimba, a Zimbabwean national, was expelled from the country, in spite of being the resident co-ordinator of United Nations operations in The Gambia, as well as the resident representative of the United Nations Development Programme. She was given an ultimatum of 48 hours to leave The Gambia because she questioned the scientific proof that the 'cure' was effective and she dared to highlight its potential to encourage high-risk behaviour (Reuters 2007; Amon 2008: 3).

Conclusion

The president's HIV/AIDS 'cure' programme is a travesty. He introduced a self-serving political agenda in the guise of healthcare, which has challenged the credibility of the national HIV/AIDS programme and exacerbated the threat of increasing HIV transmission in a country that has so far been relatively fortunate in having a low HIV prevalence. Giving 'false hope' (Starin 2007a: 294) to HIV-infected people, he has maligned their existing treatment and return to good health by insisting they abandon ARV therapies. He diverted limited resources for his 'cure'; for example, using the RVTH and Serekunda Hospital premises for screening and treatment and Department of State for Health and Social Welfare resources, staff time and skills. He manipulated social norms and values to foster belief in his 'cure'; in particular, appealing to religious beliefs and propagating fear in terms of conspiratorial accusations of racism and malfeasance on the part of external 'Western' agencies. His agenda was underpinned by coercion, specifically abuse of state security resources to quell dissent.

In the late 1990s and early years of the 2000s, Yahya Jammeh was compelled to disband his military government and establish a parliamentary democracy because of pressure ranging from economic sanctions to declining tourist numbers and domestic protests (Wiseman 1996: 932–3; 1997: 26; Edie 2000: 183; Saine 2002b: 168). However, these measures have not been applied in recent years, despite the obvious abuse of state authority and power, which has negated citizens' right to life and access to appropriate healthcare. This is the basis for the question I posed at the beginning of this chapter: Who protects the subjects when Science and the State collude to promote a counterfeit cure? There is little protection for Gambians in the face of state coercion. The question, however, should also be asked of external agencies in view of the lack of pressure from the United Nations, the World Bank, The Global Fund to Fight AIDS, Tuberculosis and Malaria (GFTAM) and WHO.

* * *

At the end of 2011, President Jammeh claimed that the HIV/AIDS programme was 'going very well' and that his critics could 'go to hell'. He has subsequently also begun a programme of treatment for 'infertility' in women.[21]

Notes

1. I adopt the word 'batch' because it is the term used by President Jammeh and is also commonly used in everyday local Gambian English to refer to serial groups of people – or example, 'the first batch of students enrolled in a course'.
2. See www.statehouse.gm/pres-rvth-board_170107.htm.
3. See www.statehouse.gm/presi-spch-hivpatient-dischrg_170607.htm.
4. See www.statehouse.gm/presi-spch-hivpatient-dischrg_170607.htm.
5. See www.statehouse.gm/presrls-president-trustfund_280207.htm.
6. See www.statehouse.gm/presi-spch-hivpatient-dischrg_170607.htm.
7. See www.statehouse.gm/editorial_210207.htm.
8. See www.statehouse.gm/swear-sosgreyjohnson_220207.htm.
9. See www.statehouse.gm/presi-hiv-rsult_180307.htm.
10. See www.statehouse.gm/images/hiv-aids-batch4/discharge_290308/result.htm.
11. See www.statehouse.gm/hiv-treatmnt-rsult_310107.htm.

12. In 2008, when the fourth batch of patients was being recruited, the president's nephew Dr Ansumana Jammeh, a traditional healer, was appointed head of the presidential medical team. It was declared that the president was still chief consultant on the project.
13. See www.statehouse.gm/hivbreakthrough-anniversary_17-01-08.htm.
14. The Taiwanese government began to provide funds for the Gambian government to pay the salaries of Cuban, Nigerian, and Egyptian doctors, and other healthcare workers in 1997 (Saine 2000b: 82; Madge 1998: 308).
15. See www.statehouse.gm/presi-spch-hivpatient-dischrg_170607.htm.
16. See www.statehouse.gm/presi-spch-hivpatient-dischrg_170607.htm.
17. This has been a theme in the president's rhetoric throughout his tenure. See Darboe (2004: 77–88) for a critical analysis of the influence of Wahhabi Islamic ideologues in The Gambia; specifically, their 'ambition of ridding Gambian Islam of all corrupting Western influences' through strategic alliance with the president.
18. In addition, there was conspicuous silence about the programme amongst other health professionals in the country, including expatriate personnel and those involved in the provision of HIV and AIDS treatment.
19. The NAS is the key institution within the NAC. It used to be located in the president's office. Then it was transferred to the Department of Health and Social Welfare but is now back in the president's office. Saihou Ceesay, the director of the NAS, and Aisha Baldeh, the Global Fund administrator, both resigned from their posts rather than be complicit with the programme. Alieu Jammeh, who was director of the NAC, was then named the new director of the NAS.
20. Prior to his death, Deyda Hydara regularly received threats from the National Intelligence Agency that was monitoring him, and was implicated in his death along with 'the Green Boys', a small vigilante militia group comprising members of the Presidential Guard and answering to Yahya Jammeh (Reporters without Borders 2008; Saine 2008a).
21. See www.bbc.co.uk/news/world-africa-16144116 and http://allafrica.com/stories/201110171842.html.

References

Amon, J. 2008. 'Dangerous Medicines: Unproven AIDS Cures and Counterfeit Antiretroviral Drugs'. *Globalization and Health* 4(5). Available at www.globalizationandhealth.com/content/4/1/5.

CPJ (Committee to Protect Journalists). 2008. 'Attacks on the Press in 2007: The Gambia'. Available at www.cpj.org/attacks07/africa07/gam07.html.

Darboe, M. 2004. 'ASR Focus: Islamism in West Africa: Gambia'. *African Studies Review* 47(2): 73–82.

Edie, C. 2000. 'Democracy in The Gambia: Past, Present and Prospects for the Future'. *Africa Development* 25(3–4): 161–99.

Feierman, S. and J. Janzen (eds). 1992. *The Social Basis of Health and Healing in Africa.* Berkeley: University of California Press.

Helman, C. 2002. *Culture, Health and Illness: An Introduction for Health Professionals.* Oxford: Butterworth-Heinemann.

Hughes, A. 2000. '"Democratisation" under the Military in The Gambia 1994–2000'. *Commonwealth and Comparative Politics* 38(3): 35–52.

IAS (International AIDS Society) and SAA (Society for AIDS in Africa). 2007. 'Joint Statement on the Gambian Government's Unproven Claim of a Cure for AIDS'. 24 April. Available at www.iasociety.org/Default.aspx?pageId=99.

International Freedom of Expression Exchange. 2007a. 'Two Journalists Fired Allegedly over Article on President, Reinstated after Minister's Plea'. 14 February. Available at www.canada.ifex.org/alerts/content/view/full/81097.

————. 2007b. 'Newspaper Journalist Fired over Article on President Jammeh's HIV/AIDS Cure'. 4 July. Available at www.ifex.org/en/content/view/full/84586.

Kandeh, J. 1996. 'What Does the "Militariat" Do When it Rules? Military Regimes: The Gambia, Sierra Leone and Liberia'. *Review of African Political Economy* 69: 387–404.

Last, M. and G. Chavunduka (eds). 1986. *The Professionalisation of African Medicine.* Manchester: Manchester University Press, Dover.

Loum, M. 2002. 'Bad Governance and Democratic Failure: A Look at Gambia's 1994 Coup'. *Civil Wars* 5(1): 145–74.

Madge, C. 1998. 'Therapeutic Landscapes of the Jola, The Gambia, West Africa'. *Health and Place* 4: 293–311.

Nyanzi, S. 2009. 'Negotiating Scripts for Meaningful Sexuality: An Ethnography of Youths in The Gambia'. Ph.D. diss. London: London School of Hygiene and Tropical Medicine at the University of London.

Nyanzi, S. and O. Bah. 2008. 'Who Protects the Subjects? The Politics of President Jammeh's HIV/AIDS Healing in The Gambia'. Paper presented at the XVII International AIDS Conference. Mexico City, Mexico.

Reporters without Borders. 2008. 'Gambia Annual Report'. Available at www.rsf.org/article.php3?id_article=25389.

Reuters. 2007. 'Gambia Expels UN Official for AIDS "Cure" Criticism'. 23 February. Available at www.alertnet.org/thenews/newsdesk/L23436011.htm.

Saine, A. 1996. 'The Coup d'État in The Gambia, 1994: The End of the First Republic'. *Armed Forces and Society* 23: 97–111.

————. 1997. 'The Presidential and National Assembly Elections in The Gambia'. *Electoral Studies* 16: 554–89.

————. 2000a. 'The Soldier-Turned-Presidential-Candidate: A Comparison of Flawed "Democratic" Transitions in Ghana and Gambia'. *Journal of Political and Military Sociology* 28: 191–209.

————. 2000b. 'The Gambia's Foreign Policy since the Coup: 1994–2000'. *Commonwealth and Comparative Politics* 38: 73–88.

————. 2002a. 'Post-Coup Politics in The Gambia'. *Journal of Democracy* 13(4): 167–72.

————. 2002b. 'The Military and Human Rights in The Gambia 1994–1999'. *Journal of Third World Studies* 19(2): 167–87.

————. 2008a. 'Presidential and National Assembly Elections, The Gambia 2006 and 2007'. *Electoral Studies* 27: 151–90.

————. 2008b. 'The Gambia's "Elected" Autocrat: Poverty, Peripherality, and Political Instability, 1994–2006'. *Armed Forces and Society* 34(3): 450–73.

Schweisfurth, M. 2002. 'Democracy and Teacher Education: Negotiating Practice in The Gambia'. *Comparative Education* 38(3): 303–14.

Shaw, M. and M. Jawo. 2000. 'Gambian Experiences with Stepping Stones: 1996–99'. *Participatory Learning and Action Notes* 37: 73–5.

Starin, D. 2007a. 'AIDS: Cures? Crisis!' *Journal of the Royal Society of Medicine* 100: 294–6.

————. 2007b. 'First-Person Dancing Lessons from God'. *Index on Censorship* 36(3): 207–14.

United Nations. 2007. 'No Evidence for Gambian AIDS "Cure"'. 16 March. Available at www.upi.com/Health_Business/Briefing/2007/03/16/un_no_evidence_for_gambian_aids_cure/8909/.

UNAIDS (Joint United Nations Programme on HIV/AIDS). 2007. 'Gambia Country Profile'. Available at www.unaids.org/en/Regions_countries/countries/Gambia. asap.

UNAIDS and WHO (World Health Organization). 2007. 'UNAIDS and WHO Underline Importance of Evidence Based Approaches to Treatment in Response to AIDS'. 16 March. Available at http://data.unaids.org/pub/pressStatement/2007/070316_gambia_statement_en.pdf.

Van der Geest, S. 1997. 'Is There a Role for Traditional Medicine in Basic Health Services in Africa? A Plea for a Community Perspective'. *Tropical Medicine and International Health* 2: 903–11.

Van der Loeff, M., R. Sarge-Njie, S. Ceesay, A. Awasana, P. Jaye, O. Sam, K.O. Jaiteh, D. Cubitt, P. Milligan and H. Whittle. 2003. 'Regional Differences in HIV Trends in The Gambia: Results from Sentinel Surveillance among Pregnant Women'. *AIDS* 17(12): 1 841–6.

WHO. 2007. 'WHO Statement on Treatment of HIV/AIDS'. 27 February. Available at www.afro.who.int/press/2007/pr20070727.html.

Wiseman, J. 1996. 'Military Rule in The Gambia: An Interim Assessment'. *Third World Quarterly* 17(5): 917–40.

————. 1997. 'Letting Yahya Jammeh off Lightly?' *Review of African Political Economy* 24(72): 265–76.

————. 1998. 'The Gambia: From Coup to Elections'. *Journal of Democracy* 9(2): 64–75.

Wiseman, J. and E. Vidler. 1995. 'The July 1994 Coup d'État in The Gambia: The End of an Era'. *The Round Table* 333: 53–65.

7

Culture, Behaviour and AIDS
in Africa

Paul Nchoji Nkwi and H. Russell Bernard

In 2007, some 33 million people worldwide were living with HIV, about 22 million of them (two-thirds of the total) in sub-Saharan Africa (UNAIDS 2008). Gains that had been made – in life expectancy, infant and child mortality and education – in the first two decades after independence began to be reversed. Those most affected by the disease were in their productive years and made up 55% of adults with HIV/AIDS. As AIDS claimed skilled labour, agricultural production was driven down, threatening food security. Increased demand for services overwhelmed the health sector. In Kenya, for example, the Human Development Index declined from 0.533 to 0.520 between 1990 and 2004 (HDR Kenya 2005: 6).

The search for causes of the epidemic has been characterised by two sets of myths. On the one hand, some African leaders have accused the West of fomenting AIDS. On the other hand, some in the West have identified various African sexual practices as facilitating or promoting the spread of HIV. The evidence against the first set of myths is well known and Gausset (2001) has made a forceful case against the second set for Tonga. In this chapter, we reinforce Gausset's position that African sexual practices are not the major problem. We make our argument on the basis of data from sub-Saharan countries and we discuss the findings of Green (2003; Green et al. 2006, 2009; Green and

Herling 2007) and others (Halperin and Epstein 2004; Shelton 2007; Kirby 2008) regarding the practice of multiple concurrent sexual partners (MCPs), which is most associated with the spread of HIV in Africa.

We stress from the outset that we do not separate the practice of MCPs from culture. The number of sexual partners considered appropriate to have in one's lifetime or concurrently is as much a cultural artefact as is the number of wives or husbands or children one is permitted or encouraged to have. We distinguish, however, between particular sexual practices and practices that are universally subject to local custom. Only some peoples practise female genital cutting (FGC) or ritualised sexual cleansing after widowhood. People everywhere can and usually do impose restrictions on the number of serial and/or concurrent sexual partners one may have. When it comes to HIV transmission, no risk is too small to ignore. Our point is that the particular sexual practices of Africans are not the major obstacle to stopping the incidence of HIV. Lowering the number of concurrent sexual partners, by contrast, is as important today in Africa as it was in San Francisco in the 1980s. The problem in San Francisco was primarily limited to homosexuals, while in Africa the HIV epidemic is a general one. The importance of lowering the number of concurrent partners, however, is the same in any epidemic of a sexually transmitted disease.

This chapter offers a critical review of the evidence of the sexual behaviours in Africa that are logically and empirically associated with the spread of HIV. The key findings are: first, having MCPs is the sexual practice most associated with the transmission of HIV; second, this practice is not unique to Africa; third, the most effective intervention programme in Africa for reducing the prevalence of HIV has been an indigenous response, 'Abstain, Be Faithful, Condomise' (widely known as ABC, begun in Uganda); and lastly, while all three components of this intervention are important, the reduction in the number of partners (the A and B of ABC) are clearly the most effective.[1]

Responses to AIDS in Africa and in the West

When the AIDS epidemic began in the 1980s, it was met with scepticism and denial in Africa. Coming in the wake of onerous structural adjustment programmes, and in the context of declining populations in the industrialised countries of the world, AIDS was seen initially by some leaders at the national and local levels in Africa as a Western ploy to stop Africans from increasing demographically. AIDS was referred to in popular circles as an 'American invention to discourage sex' (Schoepf 2004: 46) or, in its French equivalent, SIDA, as '*syndrome imaginaire pour decourager les amoureux*' (imaginary syndrome to discourage lovers) (Watney 1994: 103). This made sense to people struggling to make ends meet and without many sources of competing information, but it slowed the kind of response that was needed and the results were tragic. In South Africa alone, rejection by the government of antiretroviral (ARV) drugs for treating AIDS is estimated to have cost 330 000 lives (Chigwedere et al. 2008).

Denial of AIDS is now receding but has not disappeared. In 2007, the Archbishop of Maputo claimed that countries in Europe were exporting HIV-infected condoms to kill off Africans (McGreal 2007; see also Kalichman 2009). The response from industrialised countries to the epidemic in Africa was based on their experience with AIDS. In the West, HIV was initially spread by men who had unprotected anal sex with other men. People in San Francisco, New York and other cities with large gay populations responded quickly by educating men who have sex with men (MSM) about the importance of using condoms and, particularly in San Francisco, closing the bath houses. The rate of AIDS cases declined in those cities, creating the impression that condoms were the answer. In fact, the incidence and prevalence of AIDS went down temporarily, probably because gay men reduced the number of their sexual partners (Rotello 1997).

Indeed, by the mid-1990s, the rate of infection had rebounded and was 18.3 cases per 100 000 in San Francisco in 2009, higher than the national average of 11.2 for metropolitan areas (cities of half a million or more) and 27 cases per 100 000 in New York, more than double the national average (CDC 2009: Table 24). In the United States, the largest single cause of HIV transmission continues to be male-to-male intromissive sex. Between 2003 and 2006, the number of cases of AIDS in that population increased by 22%, from 17 678 to 21 617 in the

33 states that had confidential reporting. In the same period, new cases of AIDS as the result of high-risk heterosexual contact went down by 3%, from 4 269 to 4 152 (CDC 2006: Table 1).

Condoms and ABC

Today, the conventional package of interventions in the fight against AIDS includes treating sexually transmitted infections (STIs), providing easy access to voluntary counselling, fighting stigma through public education programmes and the distribution of condoms, along with programmes to educate people about using the device properly for each and every intro-missive sexual act in which a partner's serostatus is unknown. These efforts are certainly worth supporting, but they are, as Shelton (2007: 1811) points out, 'much more effective in conjunction with' reducing the number of sexual partners.

Between 1998 and 2002, international donors shipped an estimated 885 million condoms annually to countries in sub-Saharan Africa (Chaya, Amen and Fox 2004). This level of effort can lower HIV transmission substantially in high-risk groups – such as MSM, intravenous drug users and prostitutes – and in urban areas, such as Kampala (Kirby 2008), where networks of sexual interaction can be dense. For such relatively small and/or geographically focused groups, the problem is identifying them and reaching them with appropriate interventions. In a generalised epidemic, however, as is the case in parts of Africa, condom promotion as an intervention has failed to bring down HIV incidence or prevalence (Shelton 2006, 2007; Potts et al. 2008; Green 2003; Hearst and Chen 2004; Hogle et al. 2002; Green et al. 2009). Indeed, the promotion and distribution of condoms may produce risk compensation – a false sense of security leading some users to riskier sex than they might have had otherwise (Ahmed et al. 2001; Kajubi et al. 2005; Cassell et al. 2006; Kalichman, Eaton and Pinkerton 2007; Marrazzo 2007).

In contrast, the success of the ABC programme in Uganda – Abstain; if you can't abstain, then Be faithful; and if you can't be faithful, then Condomise – shows that programmes to delay sexual debut and reduce the number of concurrent sexual partners outside of stable unions can, along with aggressive marketing of condom use, dramatically reduce the rate of new cases of HIV (Green 2003; Green et al. 2006; Halperin and Epstein 2004; Kirby 2008). From a high of 15% in 1991, the prevalence of HIV in Uganda dropped to 4% in 2003 (Green et al. 2006: 337). However, since then Uganda has seen an increase of AIDS prevalence to 7.7% and incidence, which reached an all-time low in 2005, has begun to increase as well (Shafer et al. 2008). Nonetheless, the major lesson from Uganda is clear: ABC works, when taken seriously and supported by all levels of government.

Culture and AIDS in Africa

Support for more condoms as the primary intervention comes also, as Gausset (2001) has argued persuasively, from beliefs about African sexuality – namely, that African sexual practices increase the chance of transmission of STIs.[2]

To assess the possible role of sexual practices in Africa in the spread of HIV, Nkwi supervised a five-country study in 2003–4 for the African Population Advisory Council (Nkwi 2005). The study was funded by the United Nations Population Fund (UNFPA) through its African Social Research Program (ASRP). The study, hereafter called the ASRP study, involved ethnographic interviews with 636 local experts in Cameroon, Kenya, Malawi, Togo and Côte d'Ivoire and survey interviews with 4 802 respondents in the same countries.[3]

In developing the in-depth and survey interviews, Nkwi did a comprehensive review of the anthropological and epidemiological literature to identify the cultural practices in Africa that are logically or empirically associated with the transmission or prevention of disease, including STIs. These practices include: the use of unsterilised instruments in surgical procedures; various forms of the levirate (widow inheritance) and so-called sexual cleansing rituals; polygyny; ritualised and unprotected non-marital sex; prostitution; and non-commercial sex involving MCPs.

As we will see, some practices (such as ritualised non-marital sex) present a clear risk for the transmission of HIV. Others (polygyny and the levirate, for example) entail risk under some conditions but are protective against transmission under others. And one practice, male circumcision, is highly efficient in preventing the transmission of HIV. The extent to which any of these practices expose people to HIV is, of course, an empirical matter and requires measurement. However, all such risks are small compared to that of having unprotected sex with MCPs whose serostatus is unknown. We will have more to say about this later.

Unsterilised instruments in surgical procedures

Across Africa, various groups practise scarification, piercing and tattooing, male circumcision and FGC. Scarification, piercing and tattooing are widely practised for aesthetic purposes and as a means of ethnic identification. Among the Guiziga and Mafa peoples in Cameroon, for example, the perforations of lips and nose (for hanging rings) have been traditional symbols of ethnic identity and forms of beautification for women. Among the Samburu of Kenya, women traditionally underwent scarification of the forehead and chest to enhance their beauty.

Male circumcision is a common practice in many societies across Africa, though certainly not all. Among societies in the ASRP study, the Luo, a major ethnic group in Kenya, do not practise circumcision and traditionally initiated young men through the ritual removal of six lower teeth. Even where circumcision is the norm, the ideology that underlies this practice differs from culture to culture. In some cultures of Cameroon, for example, circumcision is performed without great ceremony, usually when a boy is between eight and ten years old or even younger. The operation is simply an exercise to remove the foreskin and enhance the sensitivity of the glans penis. Among the Samburu and Luhya in Kenya, by contrast, circumcision is part of an elaborate rite of passage from childhood to adulthood. It allows men to own and control property and prepares them for marriage. Among the Samburu, the circumcision ritual appears to take place every fifteen years.

FGC (also called female genital mutilation and female circumcision) primarily involves excision of the clitoris and excision of the labia minora but, in some groups, involves infibulation and excision of the labia majora. A common reason given for these practices by informants in the ASRP study was to prevent premarital and extramarital sex by removing the most sensitive part of the sex organ and thus prepare girls for marriage.

All of these practices involve risk of disease transmission when performed collectively or when the instruments are not sterilised between uses. The extent to which such local surgeries are a vector for HIV, however, remains to be determined. Brewer et al. (2007a, 2007b) found that adolescents in Kenya, Lesotho and Tanzania who claimed to be virgins and who had been through genital surgery (circumcision for boys, FGC for girls) were more likely than adolescents who claimed sexual experience to be HIV positive. The researchers attribute this to the transmission of HIV in local surgeries. Their finding is questioned by Adams, Trinitapoli and Poulin (2007); Westreich, Rennie and Muula (2007); and Monjok, Essien and Holmes, who conclude: 'There are no epidemiologic data associating HIV transmission with FGC' (2007: 39). Across Africa, strategic initiatives against HIV/AIDS include recommendations that new blades be used in all local surgeries and some people are even bringing their own new blades with them to ceremonies that involve cutting. Yount and Abraham (2007: 74) found that only 17% of girls who underwent an FGC operation in Kenya were exposed to a common instrument. While local surgeries are unlikely to be a major cause of HIV transmission, everyone agrees that all local surgeries need to be hygienic and safe and that continued education about the importance of using sterile instruments is vital.

This must not be read as support for the practice of FGC. Several countries have passed laws against FGC and, in some countries the practice appears to be in decline. Up to two million women per year, however, still undergo one form or another of genital cutting (for a report, see Wakabi 2007). We join the many writers over the years who have argued that FGC is an assault on the human rights of girls and women (see, for example, Eliade 1958; Nkwi 2001; Darby et al. 2007; Catania et al. 2008; Shell-Duncan 2008).

There may be little direct risk for HIV transmission in FGC practices but there may be a strong indirect risk. Yount and Abraham (2007: 80) found in Kenya that women who had been through FGC were often married young to men older than themselves and that women with older husbands were 2.65 times more likely to test positive for HIV than were women with husbands their own age or younger (11.7% of women married to older husbands, as opposed to 4.4% of women with husbands their own age or younger).

Unlike FGC, male circumcision offers some protection against the transmission of the virus. This was originally extrapolated from population-level data in sub-Saharan Africa (Weiss, Quigley and Hayes 2000). Later, three randomised controlled trials showed that male circumcision reduces the risk of contracting HIV by 50 to 60% (Auvert et al. 2005; Bailey et al. 2007; Gray et al. 2007). In fact, the three experimental studies had to be stopped for ethical reasons in order to make the intervention, circumcision, available to those in the control condition (Klausner et al. 2008: 1). It should be noted that this efficacy is for medically supervised and full circumcision. While male circumcision lessens the risk of contracting HIV, the remaining risk is substantial. In fact, circumcision, like ARV therapy, may be incorrectly perceived as protecting fully against AIDS and this may lead to risk compensation (Cassell et al. 2006). When combined with a reduction in the number of concurrent sexual partners, however, male circumcision is estimated to reduce the incidence of HIV by at least 25 to 35% (Hallett et al. 2008) and perhaps by as much as 50 to 60% (White et al. 2008).

The levirate and sexual cleansing

The levirate, or widow inheritance, is well known in Western society from the Old Testament and is practised, in one form or another, in patrilineal cultures across the world. Among the Bassa of Cameroon, for example, a married woman is considered as having entered into a permanent contract with the kin group of the husband. The death of the husband does not nullify the husband's contractual right to lineage continuity. This is achieved by transferring procreative duties to another male member of the lineage.

Among the Luhya people of Kenya, the final funeral ritual takes place 40 days after the burial of the deceased man. Relatives assemble in the house of the deceased. The widow prepares food and places it between the legs of the brother whom she has chosen (if there is more than one brother) to be her new husband. The ceremony takes place at night and ends with the consummation of the marriage the same night. The following morning, the woman shaves her pubic area, signalling a new beginning and the cutting of ties with the deceased. In the ASRP survey, 62% of Luhya respondents were against widow inheritance. However, it is still the case, as in other societies that practise the levirate, that not going through with the ceremony can stigmatise the widow and make her life difficult (Gausset 2001; Malungo 2001).

From a public health perspective, the levirate and sexual cleansing rituals for widows and widowers introduce at least one new sexual partner into each person's life, almost always without knowledge of the HIV status of either partner. Although this increases the risk of infection, it also prevents the impoverishment of widows, some of whom might otherwise be driven into prostitution. Thus, if widow inheritance does not involve the ritual practice of unsafe sex, it can inhibit rather than facilitate the transmission of HIV. In southern Zambia, as a result of the HIV epidemic, people who practise sexual cleansing of widows or widowers are seeking alternatives to the practice of penetrative sex. In a sample of 106 widowed persons there (68 women and 38 men), Malungo (2001: 375) found that 19% had been sexually cleansed, 12% had not been cleansed at all and 69% had participated in an alternative cleansing ritual that did not involve sex. This culturally appropriate change in practice was not the result of outside intervention and makes clear the importance of seeking indigenous alternatives to traditional practices.

Polygyny

Polygyny is practised among many groups across Africa. In Kenya, polygyny is legal if a man's first marriage is contracted according to customary law, but illegal if contracted after civil or Christian marriage. In Cameroon, polygyny is legal if, during the first marriage, the first wife approves of it. In Côte d'Ivoire, polygyny has been legislated against since 1964 but it is still widely practised in rural areas.

From an evolutionary perspective, polygyny is associated with high male mortality in war and high pathogen stress (Ember, Ember and Low 2007). This helps to explain the historical origins of polygyny, but it does not account for its widespread practice in Africa today. Polygyny increases lineage-level political, social and economic alliances; it functions as a child-spacing and survival strategy (especially important for women of low-income groups); it produces more total children per household in the context of high infant mortality (although Amey [2002: 84] found that it increases the individual risk of infant mortality by 60 to 70% in six West African countries); it establishes multiple affinal relationships and alliances; and it increases the potential for wealth accumulation in traditional agricultural societies.

At a cultural level, the values and beliefs that support polygyny, across religions, include a desire by women for security and a desire by men for increased social status and for a measure of immortality through increased procreation. One ASRP informant in Butere, Kenya had this to say: 'My first wife had only three children, so I decided to marry a second wife to have more children. Also my second wife did not give me a son and she had only daughters and that is why I have three wives'.

In a newscast on 16 March 2003, a Cameroon national television journalist interviewed a popular musician known as Papillion about the content and meaning of one of his songs. Papillon said: '*Vous savez, tout homme normal doit avoir un deuxième bureau*' (You know, every man ought to have a mistress). The reference in French is to a 'second office', meaning a woman (or more than one woman), besides his wife or wives, with whom a man shares his life regularly. Many married male informants who were interviewed in the ASRP study provided similar explanations to the existence of the practice.

With regard to HIV, if the men in polygynous unions sleep around and do not use condoms in every penetrative sexual act, this practice places all women in the household at risk of HIV, along with the infants of those women through placental and breast milk transfer of the virus.

Polygyny, however, is not a channel for STIs if the partners are faithful to one another – a practice known as 'zero grazing' across Anglophone Africa.[4] In many sub-Saharan societies, however, where polygyny is normative, wives are expected to be faithful whereas husbands are expected or even encouraged to have extramarital affairs. Postpartum sexual abstinence for women is understood in many cultures as protecting the life and health of the mother and child but it also then becomes a rationale for polygyny and for extramarital sex for men (Mitsunaga et al. 2005: 478; Ali and Cleland 2001).

As a cultural practice, polygyny appears to be under pressure in Africa. In the 1970s, 33% of households in the Kisii region of western Kenya were polygynous. By the late 1990s, less than 10% of households in the same region were polygynous (Silberschmidt 2001: 662). Between 1990 and 2003 in Nigeria, the percentage of married women in polygynous unions fell from 41 to 36% (Mitsunaga et al. 2005: 479). Increasing poverty on the continent means that the cost of maintaining a polygynous household has become prohibitive for many men and, as women enter the workforce, the latter no longer need to be part of polygynous households to secure their old age. Young men and women in Africa increasingly find polygyny unnecessary and undesirable and the practice will likely erode over time, though later among some groups than others. Polygyny is nominally disapproved of across the ASRP study sites. It is rejected as an ideal form of marriage in Cameroon (79.5%), Côte d'Ivoire (80.4%), Togo (81.3%), Kenya (81%) and Malawi (45%).

As of 2005, the risk of HIV in Uganda was no higher in polygynous households than in monogamous ones (Ministry of Health and ORC Macro 2006: 105). The decline of formal polygyny, however, has been found in Uganda and in other African countries to be accompanied by informal polygyny – that is, a group of co-wives in physically separate households, who are not formally connected to one another and who may not even know one another. Under these conditions, as Parikh (2007: 1 205) found, 'women have no reason not to have multiple male partners . . . to provide additional economic and affective support, thus intensifying HIV risk for all sexual partners'.

Ritualised non-marital sex

Across Africa, some ethnic groups ritualise premarital and extramarital sex. A practice that has received particular attention is the ritualised sexual initiation of pubescent and prepubescent girls. Among the Chewa and Yao ethnic groups of Malawi, the practice, known as *fisi* (hyena, in the local language), involves sexual intercourse between an adult man and adolescent girls at the end of an initiation ceremony (Kamwendo and Kamowa 1999: 168).

Data from the ASRP study show that the ritual takes three forms. In the first, girls who have reached puberty are secluded for several weeks and given instruction on sex and reproduction and on the role that men and women play in the process. Three to four male instructors will have sexual intercourse with the girls at the close of the period of seclusion. According to local belief, the process enhances and guarantees the fertility of the girls. When a man marries a woman, he expects her to have undergone the ritual. As the local saying goes: 'No *fisi*, no husband.' A second form of *fisi* can be referred to as consensual adultery. If a woman does not become pregnant, despite having undergone the *fisi* ritual, the husband can hire another man to have sex with his wife to impregnate her. Finally, in a third form of *fisi* known as *kulongosola mwana* (taking the baby back), another man has sex with the nursing mother before the husband resumes sexual relations with his wife (Sungani 1998). The HIV/AIDS status of the men who play the *fisi* role is not known, thereby exposing girls and married women to an unmeasured risk of infection.

In Kenya, some funeral rituals are said to involve sexual licence. Among the Luhya people of Wanga, for example the commemoration of the dead (*lung'anyo*, or revisiting the shadow of the dead) is based on the idea that the spirit of the deceased person needs to be provided with a peaceful entry into the spirit world. The ritual facilitates that process by cleansing the living from any evils and stigma associated with the dead and also commemorates and appeases the dead. The ceremony takes place a month after a person's death and involves all married members of the community. It consists of eating, drinking and dancing, and culminates in sexual intercourse among those assembled. Pregnancies following this ritual are believed to be the reincarnation of the deceased. A male informant in the ASRP study described the ceremony as follows:

> During the night, the dead person is supposed to be named and the naming is only supposed to be done by members of the family and hence the presence of the *abakoko*. As the festivity gathers momentum, people start picking their mates randomly, this culminates into sexual encounters. You just chose whomever you come into contact with. People say today is *omuhula* (the naming of the dead). So everybody attempts to conceive so that they can be able to name the dead. Nobody is supposed to refuse these advances because everyone knows the essence of assembling at the deceased's home. People look forward to this ceremony because of the sexual activities (Nkwi 2005).

As one would expect, the use of condoms during this ceremony is forbidden because it defeats the ideology of reincarnation through sexual intercourse. The multiple acts of sex create the opportunity for the spread of HIV.

Among the Samburus of northern Kenya, the sexual initiation of young girls and the participation of adult men (called *morans*) in the tourist trade for sex produces a high risk of exposure to HIV/AIDS. From ethnographic data in the ASRP study, circumcised Samburu men are theoretically entitled to sex with any available woman. Young men who fall in love express their feelings by adorning a young girl with beads and showering her with gifts. This beading culture has come to symbolise Kenya for many tourists and Samburu men have become the object of attraction for some female tourists who pay to have sex with them. The Samburu believe that sperm are vital for creating children and that having sex with a condom is tantamount to denying life to come into being; their liaisons with tourist women are reported to be typically without condoms. One *moran* informant in the ASRP study said this about women tourists seeking sex:

> When a white woman sees you at the park they tell you I love
> you and I want you now. You give her two shots [sex] and you
> get Ksh.20, 000. *Mzungu* (Europeans) like sex; they also like the
> way we walk, the way we dress and our disposition . . . they
> need men like Samburu *morans* who eat herbs, meat and milk
> and they give us money so we are all satisfied but sometimes it
> adds AIDS (Nkwi 2005).

If the *morans* return to their home villages and engage in sex with
unmarried girls, this creates more opportunities for HIV infection.

The treatment of infertility sometimes leads to so-called therapeutic
sex between healers and their patients. This is reported for some ethnic
groups of north Cameroon. In this case, an infertile female patient
submits to the healer in the belief that this will help her recover her
fertility. The risk of infection increases with the number of patients
(see Runganga, Sundby and Aggleton [2001] for a report of this in
Zimbabwe).

Multiple concurrent sexual partners and poverty

Finally, the most important vehicle, by far, for the spread of HIV/
AIDS is the practice of MCPs. Morris and Kretzschmar (1997, 2000)
modelled the rate at which HIV spreads in a population characterised
by serial monogamy compared to one in which people have multiple
concurrent partners.[5] In Uganda, the observed level of concurrency in
1994 resulted in 26% more infections after five years than would have
been the case under serial monogamy (Morris and Kretzschmar 2000:
124).[6] Empirical studies have corroborated the importance of partner
reduction in holding back the spread of HIV. While the use of condoms
and voluntary testing may have contributed in part, the decline in
prevalence of HIV in Uganda (from 15% in the early 1990s to 4% in
2003) was fundamentally the result of behaviour change – in particular,
the reduction in the number of sexual partners (Stoneburner and Low-
Beer 2004; Green et al. 2006).[7]

One source of concurrent partners is commercial, transactional
sex, mostly by women. The link between poverty, commercial sex and
HIV transmission is obvious and well documented (see, for example,

Pisani 2008). Another source of concurrent partners, however, is non-commercial, transactional sex – again, mostly by young women but sometimes by young men. Poverty plays a strong role in these transactions, but there may be other causes as well. Data from the ASRP study, for example, show that young women are increasingly engaged in sexual relations with so-called 'sugar daddies', much older men, who take care of immediate financial needs, such as school fees, rent and food. In Cameroon, the girls call these married men *cou plié* or folded necks or *mbomas* and the transactional sex with them is considered temporary. Young women in the ASRP study reported that during these relationships they could not refuse to have unprotected sexual intercourse. Some of the young women with 'sugar daddies' reported also having a regular boyfriend of their own age, who may or may not have known about the 'sugar daddy'.

On the other hand, young women in the ASRP study also reported having several sexual partners of their own age. They justified this in terms of the search for new sexual experiences and for emotional security – that is, a need to have a 'standby partner . . . someone on whom you can rely in case you get beaten by your lover'. In any of these multi-partner relations, whether based on economic need or for other reasons, the risk of HIV increases for everyone in the network if one of the partners is an older 'sugar daddy'.[8]

Poverty supports the cultural practice of marrying adolescent girls to older men, as families turn their young daughters into economic assets. This increases the risk among young girls for exposure to HIV if the older husbands are already infected with the virus or if the husbands have other, concurrent partners. In urban Zambia and Kenya, Clark (2004) found HIV prevalence higher among married adolescent girls, fifteen to nineteen years of age, than among their unmarried counterparts. Furthermore, in these unions, the husbands (typically much older than the girls) were three times more likely to be HIV positive than were the boyfriends of unmarried girls, despite the fact that the reported number of sexual partners for unmarried girls in the study ranged from 0 to 21, whereas the under-twenty married women typically have just one partner (Clark 2004: 155).

Clark's findings corroborate those of Kelly et al. (2003), who found that sexually active, unmarried adolescent females (fifteen to nineteen years old) in Uganda were significantly less likely to be infected with HIV than were their married counterparts. Among married women in this age group whose partners were at least ten years older than them, the risk of contracting HIV was twice that of women whose partners were no more than four years their senior. Older husbands are increasingly likely to be infected and to pass that infection on to their younger wives (Kelly et al. 2003: 446).

In Kisumu, Kenya and in Ndola, Zambia, Glynn et al. found that 'despite the age gap at marriage and the young age at marriage for women, almost twice as many women as men were estimated to be HIV-infected at the time of their first marriage' (2003: 532). This may be because of earlier sexual debut among women and the higher prevalence of male-to-female transmission of HIV than female-to-male transmission (Hugonnet et al. 2002). Over time, however, Glynn et al. found that 'at least one quarter of HIV-positive men [were] infected from extramarital partnerships' (2003: 530).

In other words, women as well as men can bring HIV infection home. The self-reported rate of extramarital sex for women in Africa, relative to that for men, is low but may be underreported. According to the Global Program on AIDS, about 6% of women in Africa reported extramarital sex in 1995 compared to about 16% of men (Kirby 2008: 55). In a study of five African countries, De Walque (2007: 505) found that women alone were infected in 30 to 40% of infected couples. This points either to premarital infection by women or to extramarital sex by women as the unreported source of HIV transmission.

With regard to premarital infection, Bongaarts found a strong association in 33 sub-Saharan countries 'between a high average age at marriage and a long period of premarital intercourse during which partner changes are relatively common and facilitate the spread of HIV' (2007: 73). With regard to extramarital infection, Tawfik and Watkins (2007) found that rural women and men in Malawi, especially women, recognised that women take extramarital lovers for reasons other than for escaping poverty: to obtain consumer goods that their husbands cannot provide, for revenge against the infidelities of their husbands and for passion. Women in the rural Balaka province of Malawi, say Tawfik and Watkins, are not the 'poor, powerless, and passionless' beings they are made out to be in the narrative of the Western AIDS-fighting establishment (2007: 1091).

Finally, while many infectious diseases are the consequences of poverty, the risk of contracting HIV actually increases with wealth across sub-Saharan Africa. In a study of families in eight countries across sub-Saharan Africa, the prevalence of HIV was, in every case, 'higher among adults belonging to the wealthiest 20% of households than among those from the poorest 20%' (Mishra et al. 2007: S20). In all eight countries, the wealthier men and women were more likely to use condoms and the wealthier men were more likely to be circumcised (i.e. factors which inhibit the spread of HIV). However, in every country but one (Tanzania), wealthier men report having more sexual partners (both lifetime and in the last year) and more casual (that is, non-regular) partners than do poorer men. These findings, based on large samples and linked to blood tests for HIV (S18), corroborate earlier studies that were based on population-level statistics (O'Farrell 2001; Shelton, Cassell and Adetunji 2005) that the risk of HIV increases with wealth in Africa.

Conclusion

As we develop interventions against HIV/AIDS, we should ask first: What practices increase the risk of HIV transmission and what practices lower that risk and second, how can we help discourage the former and promote the latter? Culturally appropriate interventions for eliminating FGC and for eliminating unprotected ritual sex are important, as are education programmes to ensure the use of sterile instruments in all instances of local surgery. But these and other African cultural practices are not the major obstacles to lowering the prevalence of HIV.

The evidence is now abundant that first, reducing the number of concurrent sexual partners (the combination of A and B in ABC) outside stable unions was key to the success of efforts in Uganda to reduce the prevalence of HIV (Green 2003; Halperin and Epstein 2004; Kirby 2008) and second, that recent successes in Kenya (Green and Herling 2007: 27) and Zimbabwe (Gregson et al. 2006) are also the result of partner reduction.

All societies rely mainly on the internalisation of norms to regulate behaviour. State-level societies do not have enough police to keep people from killing one another, much less to keep them from running red lights. Even in small-scale societies, there are not enough eyes to watch everyone all the time, although informal social-control mechanisms in those societies have a better chance of working because people tend to remain in face-to-face contact throughout their lives. Policing everyone's sexual behaviour is impossible and handing out millions of condoms will not, by itself, solve the problem of HIV transmission.

We have a chance to combat AIDS by creating norms that prevent people from engaging in behaviours that carry a high risk of infection. This was clearly done in Uganda and other countries with culturally sensitive programmes that not only challenged or discouraged cultural practices deemed to increase risk of HIV transmission (for example, widow inheritance), but also built upon and reinforced practices, such as delaying sexual debut, that decrease the risk of HIV transmission. Both ways to deal with culture and HIV risk merit our closest attention.

Notes

1. We are grateful to Edward Green, Allison Herling, and Clarence Gravlee for helpful suggestions on drafts of this chapter.
2. The practice of 'dry sex', for example, involves removing the lubricating fluids in the vagina by douching and drying. It increases friction during coitus but apparently does not increase the risk of HIV (Myer et al. 2005, 2006).
3. The researchers who collaborated in data collection and analysis were: Socpa Antoine (Cameroon), Kofi Nguessan (Cote d'Ivoire), Judith Karogo (Kenya), Wycliffe Masoo (Malawi), and Adade Messan (Togo).
4. The phrase 'zero grazing' appears to have been introduced by Samuel Ikwaras Okware, the commissioner for health services in Uganda in 1987 when that country launched its ABC programme against AIDS.
5. For more on modelling of the effect of MCP, see Anderson (1996, 1999), Hudson (1993), and Watts and May (1992).

6. See Parikh (2007) for a detailed account of this difference in expectations in Uganda.
7. See Mah and Halperin (2008) for a review of the evidence on the effect of MCP on HIV epidemics in Africa.
8. The phenomenon of sugar mammies, older, working, married or unmarried women who engage in semi-permanent, discreet sexual relations with young boys in return for material support, was earlier reported by Silberschmidt (2001: 665) and was also found in the ASRP study.

References

Adams, J., J. Trinitapoli and M. Poulin. 2007. 'Response to Brewer et al.: Male and female Circumcision Associated with Prevalent HIV Infection in Virgins and Adolescents in Kenya, Lesotho, and Tanzania'. *Annals of Epidemiology* 17: 923–5.

Ahmed, S., T. Lutalo, M. Mawer, D. Serwadda, N. Sewankambo, F. Nalugoda, F. Makumbi, F. Wabwire-Mangen, N. Kiwanuka, G. Kigozi, M. Kiddaguvu and R. Gray. 2001. 'HIV Incidence and Sexually Transmitted Disease Prevalence Associated with Condom Use: A Population Study in Rakai, Uganda'. *AIDS* 15: 2 171–9.

Ali, M. and J. Cleland. 2001. 'The Link between Postnatal Abstinence and Extramarital Sex in Côte d'Ivoire'. *Studies in Family Planning* 32: 214–19.

Amey, F. 2002. 'Polygyny and Child Survival in West Africa'. *Social Biology* 49(1–2): 74–89.

Anderson, R. 1996. 'The Spread of HIV and Sexual Mixing Patterns'. In J. Mann and D. Tarantola (eds). *AIDS in the World II*. New York: Oxford University Press: 71–86.

———. 1999. 'Transmission Dynamics of Sexually Transmitted Infections'. In K. Holmes, P. Sparling and P-A. Mardh (eds). *Sexually Transmitted Diseases*. 3rd ed. New York: McGraw-Hill: 25–37.

Auvert, B., D. Taljaard, E. Lagarde, J. Sobngwi-Tambekou, R. Sitta and A. Puren. 2005. 'Randomized, Controlled Intervention Trial of Male Circumcision for Reduction of HIV Infection Risk: The ANRS 1265 Trial'. *PLoS Med* 2(11). Available at www.plosmedicine.org/article/info:doi/10.1371/journal.pmed. 0020298.

Bailey, R.C., S. Moses, C.B. Parker, K. Agot, I. Maclean, J.N. Krieger, C.F.M. Williams, R.T. Campbell and J.O. Ndinya-Achola. 2007. 'Male Circumcision for HIV Prevention in Young Men in Kisumu, Kenya: A Randomised Controlled Trial'. *Lancet* 369(9562): 643–56.

Bongaarts, J. 2007. 'Late Marriage and the HIV Epidemic in sub-Saharan Africa'. *Population Studies* 61: 73–83.

Brewer, D., J. Potterat, M. Roberts and S. Brody. 2007a. 'Male and Female Circumcision Associated with Prevalent HIV Infection in Virgins and Adolescents in Kenya, Lesotho, and Tanzania'. *Annals of Epidemiology* 17: 217–26.

————. 2007b. 'Circumcision-Related HIV Risk and the Unknown Mechanism of Effect in the Male Circumcision Trials'. *Annals of Epidemiology* 17: 928–9.

Cassell, M., D. Halperin, J. Shelton and D. Stanton. 2006. 'Risk Compensation: The Achilles' Heel of Innovation in HIV Prevention?' *British Medical Journal* 332: 605–7. Available at www.bmj.com/cgi/content/full/332/7541/605.

Catania, L., O. Abdulcadir, V. Puppo, J. Bverde, J. Abdulcadir and D. Abdulcadir. 2008. 'Pleasure and Orgasm in Women with Female Genital Mutilation/Cutting (FGM/C)'. *Journal of Sexual Medicine* 4: 1666–78.

CDC (Center for Disease Control and Prevention). 2006. 'Cases of HIV Infection and AIDS in the United States and Dependent Areas, 2006'. Available at www. cdc.gov/hiv/surveillance/resources/reports/2006report/.

————. 2009. 'Diagnoses of HIV Infection and AIDS in the United States and Dependent Areas, 2009'. Available at www.cdc.gov/hiv/surveillance/resources/reports/2009report/.

Chaya, N., K. Amen and M. Fox. 2004. 'Condoms Count: Meeting the Need in the Era of HIV/AIDS: 2004 Data Update'. Population Action International. Available at www.populationaction.org/Publications/Reports/Condoms_Count/2004_Data_Update.pdf.

Chigwedere, P., G. Seage III, S. Gruskin, T-H. Lee and M. Essex. 2008. 'Estimating the Lost Benefits of Antiretroviral Drug Use in South Africa'. *Journal of Acquired Immune Deficiency Syndromes* 49: 410–15.

Clark, S. 2004. 'Early Marriage and HIV Risks in sub-Saharan Africa'. *Studies in Family Planning* 35: 149–60.

Darby, R., J. Svoboda, T. Hobbes, A. Rahman and N. Toubia. 2007. 'A Rose by Any Other Name? Rethinking the Similarities and Differences between Male and Female Genital Cutting'. *Medical Anthropology Quarterly* 21: 301–23.

De Walque, D. 2007. 'Sero-Discordant Couples in Five Countries: Implications for Prevention Strategies'. *Population and Development Review* 33: 501–23.

Eliade, M. 1958. *Rites and Symbols of Initiation: The Mysteries of Birth and Rebirth.* London: Harper Torchbooks.

Ember, M., C. Ember and B. Low. 2007. 'Comparing Explanations of Polygyny'. *Cross-Cultural Research* 41: 428–40.

Gausset, Q. 2001. 'AIDS and Cultural Practices in Africa: The Case of the Tonga (Zambia)'. *Social Science and Medicine* 52: 509–18.

Glynn, J., M. Caraël, A. Buvé, R. Musonda, M. Kahindo and Study Group on the Heterogeneity of HIV Epidemics in African Cities. 2003. 'HIV Risk in Relation to Marriage in Areas with High Prevalence of HIV Infection'. *Journal of Acquired Immune Deficiency Syndromes* 35: 526–35.

Gray, R., G. Kigozi, D. Serwadda, F. Makumbi, S. Watya, F. Nalugoda, N. Niwanuka, L. Moulton, M. Chaudhary, M. Chen, N. Sewankambo, F. Wabwire-Mangen, M. Bacon, C. Williams, P. Opendi, S. Reynolds, O. Laeyendecker, T. Quinn and M. Wawer. 2007. 'Male Circumcision for HIV Prevention in Men in Rakai, Uganda: A Randomised Trial'. *Lancet* 369(9 562): 657–66.

Green, E. 2003. *Rethinking AIDS Prevention: Learning from Successes in Developing Countries*. Westport: Praeger.

Green, E., D. Halperin, V. Nantulya and J. Hogle. 2006. 'Uganda's HIV Prevention Success: The Role of Sexual Behaviour Change and the National Response'. *AIDS and Behaviour* 10: 335–46.

Green, E. and A. Herling. 2007. 'The ABC Approach to Preventing the Sexual Transmission of HIV: Common Questions and Answers'. Christian Connection for International Health. Available at www.ccih.org/resources/ABCplus/Green &Herling_ABC_Approach_2007.pdf.

Green, E., T. Mah, A. Ruark and N. Hearst. 2009. 'A Framework of Sexual Partnerships: Risks and Implications for HIV Prevention in Africa'. *Studies in Family Planning* 40(1): 63–70.

Gregson, S., G. Garnett, C. Nyamukapa, T. Hallett, J. Lewis, P. Mason, S. Chandiwana and R. Anderson. 2006. 'HIV Decline Associated with Behavior Change in Eastern Zimbabwe'. *Science* 3: 664–6.

Hallett, T., K. Singh, J. Smith, R. White, L. Abu-Raddad and G. Garnett. 2008. 'Understanding the Impact of Male Circumcision Interventions on the Spread of HIV in Southern Africa'. *PLoS ONE* 3(5): e2212: 1–9.

Halperin, D. and H. Epstein. 2004. 'Concurrent Sexual Partnerships Help to Explain Africa's High HIV Prevalence: Implications for Prevention'. *Lancet* 363(9 428): 4–6.

HDR (Human Development Report), Kenya. 2005. 'Linking Industrialization with Human Development'. United Nations Development Program. Available at http://hdr.undp.org/en/reports/nationalreports/africa/kenya/kenya_2005_en.pdf.

Hearst, N. and S. Chen. 2004. 'Condom Promotion for AIDS Prevention: Is it Working?' *Studies in Family Planning* 35: 39–47.

Hogle, J., A. Green, V. Natulya, R. Stoneburner and J. Stover. 2002. 'What Happened in Uganda? Declining HIV Prevalence, Behavior Change, and the National Response'. Available at www.usaid.gov/our_work/global_health/aids/Countries/africa/uganda_report.pdf.

Hudson, C.P. 1993. 'Concurrent Partnerships Could Cause AIDS Epidemics'. *International Journal of STD and AIDS* 4: 249–53.

Hugonnet, S., F. Mosha, J. Todd, K. Mugeye, A. Klokke, L. Ndeki, D. Ross, H. Grosskurth and R. Hays. 2002. 'Incidence of HIV Infection in Stable Sexual Partnerships: A Retrospective Cohort Study of 1 802 Couples in Mwanza Region, Tanzania'. *Journal of Acquired Immune Deficiency Syndromes* 30: 73–80.

Kajubi P., M. Kamya, S. Kamya, S. Chen, W. McFarland and N. Hearst. 2005. 'Increasing Condom Use without Reducing HIV Risk: Results of a Controlled Community Trial in Uganda'. *Journal of Acquired Immune Deficiency Syndromes* 40(1): 77–82.

Kalichman, S. 2009. *Denying AIDS: Conspiracy Theories, Pseudoscience, and Human Tragedy*. New York: Copernicus Books.

Kalichman, S., L. Eaton and S. Pinkerton. 2007. 'Circumcision for HIV Prevention: Failure to Fully Account for Behavioral Risk Compensation'. *PLoS Med* 4(3): e138. Available at www.plosmedicine.org/article/info:doi/10.1371/journal. pmed.0040138.

Kamwendo, G. and O. Kamowa. 1999. 'HIV/AIDS and a Return to Traditional Cultural Practices in Malawi'. In K.R. Hope (ed.). *AIDS and Development in Africa*. New York: Haworth Press: 165–76.

Kelly, R., R. Gray, N. Sewankambo, D. Serwadda, F. Wabwire-Mangen, T. Lutalo and M. Wawer. 2003. 'Age Differences in Sexual Partners and Risk of HIV-1 Infection in Rural Uganda'. *Journal of Acquired Immune Deficiency Syndromes* 32: 446–51.

Kirby, D. 2008. *Success in Uganda: A History of Uganda's Successful Campaign to Decrease HIV Prevalence in the Early 1990s*. Scotts Valley, CA: ETR Associates. Available at www.etr.org/uganda.

Klausner, J., R. Wamai, K. Bowa, A. Kwango, J. Kagimba and D. Halperin. 2008. 'Is Male Circumcision As Good As the HIV Vaccine We've Been Waiting for?' *Future HIV Therapy* 2: 1–7.

Mah, T. and D. Halperin. 2008. 'Concurrent Sexual Partnerships and the HIV Epidemics in Africa: Evidence to Move Forward'. *AIDS and Behavior* 14: 11–16.

Malungo, J.R.S. 2001. 'Sexual Cleansing (*Kusalazya*) and Levirate Marriage (*Kunjilila mung'anda*) in the Era of AIDS: Changes in Perceptions and Practices in Zambia'. *Social Science and Medicine* 53: 371–82.

Marrazzo, J. 2007. 'Syphilis and Other Sexually Transmitted Diseases in HIV Infection'. *Topics in HIV Medicine* 15(1): 11–16.

McGreal, C. 2007. 'HIV-Infected Condoms Sent to Kill Africans, Claims Archbishop'. *The Guardian*, 26 September. Available at www.guardian.co.uk/world/2007/ sep/27/aids.international.

Ministry of Health (Uganda) and ORC Macro. 2006. 'Uganda HIV/AIDS Sero-Behavioural Survey 2004–2005'. Ministry of Health and ORC Macro, Calverton, Maryland.

Mishra, V., S. Assche, R. Greener, M. Vaessen, R. Hong, P. Ghys, J. Boerma, A. Van Assche, S. Khan and R. Rutstein. 2007. 'HIV Infection Does Not Disproportionately Affect the Poorer in Sub-Saharan Africa'. *AIDS* 2(Supplement 7): S17–S28.

Mitsunaga, T., A. Powell, N. Heard and U. Larsen. 2005. 'Extramarital Sex among Nigerian Men: Polygyny and Other Risk Factors'. *Journal of Acquired Immune Deficiency Syndromes* 39: 478–87.

Monjok, E., E. Essien and L. Holmes Jr. 2007. 'Female Genital Mutilation: Potential for HIV Transmission in Sub-Saharan Africa and Prospect for Epidemiologic Investigation and Intervention'. *African Journal of Reproductive Health* 11: 33–42.

Morris, M. and M. Kretzschmar. 1997. 'Concurrent Partnerships and the Spread of HIV'. *AIDS* 11: 641–8.

——. 2000. 'A Microsimulation Study of the Effect of Concurrent Partnerships on the Spread of HIV in Uganda'. *Mathematical Population Studies* 8: 109–33.

Myer, L., L. Denny, M. de Souza, T. Wright Jr and L. Kuhn. 2006. 'Distinguishing the Temporal Association between Women's Intravaginal Practices and Risk of Human Immunodeficiency Virus Infection: A Prospective Study of South African Women'. *American Journal of Epidemiology* 163: 552–60.

Myer, L., L. Kuhn, Z. Stein, T. Wright and L. Denny. 2005. 'Intravaginal Practices, Bacterial Vaginosis, and Women's Susceptibility to HIV Infection: Epidemiological Evidence and Biological Mechanisms'. *Lancet* 5: 786–94.

Nkwi, P. 2001. 'Demographic Behaviour and Its Socio-Cultural Context in Cameroon'. In S. Syed (ed.). *Cultures of Populations: Population Dynamics and Sustainable Development*. Hamburg: UNESCO HQ Social Sciences: 25–70. Available at http://unesdoc.unesco.org/images/0012/001240/124028eo.pdf.

——. 2005. 'The Impact of Cultural Practices on the Spread of HIV/AIDS: An Anthropological Study of Selected Countries in Sub-Saharan Africa'. *Discovery and Innovation* 17(Special Issue): 21–35.

O'Farrell, N. 2001. 'Poverty and HIV in Sub-Saharan Africa'. *Lancet* 357(9 256): 636–7.

Parikh, S. 2007. 'The Political Economy of Marriage and HIV: The ABC Approach, "Safe" Infidelity, and Managing Moral Risk in Uganda'. *American Journal of Public Health* 97: 1198–208.

Pisani, E. 2008. *The Wisdom of Whores: Bureaucrats, Brothels, and the Business of AIDS*. New York: Norton.

Potts, M., D. Halperin, D. Kirby, A. Swidler, E. Marseille, J. Klausner, N. Hearst, R. Wamai, J. Kahn and J. Walsh. 2008. 'Reassessing HIV Prevention'. *Science* 320(5 877): 749–50.

Rotello, G. 1997. *Sexual Ecology: AIDS and the Destiny of Gay Men*. New York: Dutton.

Runganga, A., J. Sundby and P. Aggleton. 2001. 'Culture Identity and Reproductive Failure in Zimbabwe'. *Sexualities* 4: 315–32.

Schoepf, B. 2004. 'AIDS'. In D. Nugent and J. Vincent (eds). *A Companion to the Anthropology of Politics*. Malden: Blackwell: 37–54.

Shafer, L., S. Biraro, J. Nakiyingi-Miiro, A. Kamali, D. Ssematimba, J. Ouma, A. Ojwiya, P. Hughes, L. van der Paal, J. Whitworth, A. Opio and H. Grosskurth. 2008. 'HIV Prevalence and Incidence Are No Longer Falling in Southwest Uganda: Evidence from a Rural Population Cohort 1989–2005'. *AIDS* 22: 1 641–9.

Shell-Duncan, B. 2008. 'From Health to Human Rights: Female Genital Cutting and the Politics of Intervention'. *American Anthropologist* 110: 225–36.

Shelton, J. 2006. 'Confessions of a Condom Lover'. *Lancet* 368(9 551): 1947–9.

———. 2007. 'Ten Myths and One Truth about Generalised HIV Epidemics'. *Lancet* 370(9602): 1809–11.

Shelton, J., M. Cassell and J. Adetunji. 2005. 'Is Poverty or Wealth at the Root of HIV?' *Lancet* 366(9 491): 1057–8.

Silberschmidt, M. 2001. 'Disempowerment of Men in Rural and Urban East Africa: Implications for Male Identity and Sexual Behaviour'. *World Development* 4: 657–71.

Stoneburner, R. and D. Low-Beer. 2004. 'Population-Level HIV Declines and Behavioral Risk Avoidance in Uganda'. *Science* 304: 714–18.

Sungani, L. 1998. 'Chiputu or Simba: Initiation for Young Girls'. B.A. dissertation paper, Theology Department, Chancellor College, Zomba.

Tawfik, L. and S. Watkins. 2007. 'Sex in Geneva, Sex in Lilongwe, and Sex in Balaka'. *Social Science and Medicine* 64: 1090–101.

UNAIDS (Joint United Nations Programme on HIV/AIDS). 2008. 'A Global View of HIV Infection'. Map. Available at http://data.unaids.org/pub/GlobalReport/2008/GR08_2007_HIVPrevWallMap_GR08_en.jpg.

Wakabi, W. 2007. 'Africa Battles to Make Female Genital Mutilation History'. *Lancet* 369(9 567): 1069–70.

Watney, S. 1994. *Practices of Freedom: Selected Writings on HIV/AIDS*. Durham: Duke University Press.

Watts, C. and R. May. 1992. 'The Influence of Concurrent Partnerships on the Dynamics of HIV/AIDS'. *Mathematical Biosciences* 108: 89–104.

Weiss, H., M. Quigley and R. Hayes. 2000. 'Male Circumcision and Risk of HIV Infection in Sub-Saharan Africa: A Systematic Review and Meta-Analysis'. *AIDS* 14: 2361–70.

Westreich, D., S. Rennie and A. Muula. 2007. 'Comments on Brewer et al.: Male and Female Circumcision Associated with Prevalent HIV Infection in Virgins and Adolescents in Kenya, Lesotho, and Tanzania'. *Annals of Epidemiology* 17: 926–7.

White, R., J. Glynn, K. Orroth, E. Freeman, R. Bakker, H. Weiss, L. Kumaranayake, J. Dik, F. Habbema, A. Buvé and R. Hayes. 2008. 'Male Circumcision for HIV Prevention in Sub-Saharan Africa: Who, What and When?' *AIDS* 22: 1841–50.

Yount, K. and B. Abraham. 2007. 'Female Genital Cutting and HIV/AIDS among Kenyan Women'. *Studies in Family Planning* 38: 73–88.

8

Sexuality and Rights

Men Who Have Sex with Men in Addis Ababa, Ethiopia

Getnet Tadele

Research on sexuality has established the presence of homosexuality in about fifty African societies, despite widespread popular and religious discourse claiming that homosexuality is not an 'African' phenomenon (Parker, Khan and Aggleton 1998; Niang et al. 2003; Murray and Roscoe 1998). This chapter stems from a study on the sexual lives of men who have sex with men (MSM) in Addis Ababa, Ethiopia, where homosexuality is illegal and there is some policing by the state. The results indicate that homosexuality exists in Ethiopian society and suggest that there is a flourishing underground commercial sex trade in Addis Ababa. However, informants report high levels of prejudice and internalised stigma. Using a (sexual) citizenship and rights framework, this chapter argues for the need to create space for a discussion of the various types of sexual relationships in Ethiopia. The results also highlight that current efforts aimed at preventing the spread of HIV are not addressing some so-called high-risk behaviours and interventions could benefit from an approach that addresses different sexual practices and identities. I also interrogate the dual role of the state as both agency of social justice and vehicle of domination in the area of sexuality and how the regime of disciplining and monitoring of the body in Ethiopia has affected MSM's sexuality and the risk of exposure to HIV/AIDS.

With varying degrees of prevalence, different forms of sexual relationships take place in virtually all societies. While heterosexuality is the most upheld sexual norm in most societies, homosexuality is also common (Tesfaye 1988). Unpacking the term homosexuality, there are specific identities such as lesbian, gay, bisexual and transgender. In many non-Western societies, most people do not recognise themselves as heterosexual, gay, bisexual, lesbian, or transgender as these subjective sexual identities are peculiar to the Western world.

There is an increasing recognition that the relation between sexual identity and sexual behaviour is fluid and that classifications such as heterosexual, homosexual, gay, queer and bisexual are social constructs not clearly related to sexual behaviour (Weeks 1995; Parker and Gagnon 1995). Efforts to prevent the spread of HIV/AIDS among those who do not identify themselves in social identities motivated scholars and activists to come up with another label: Men who have sex with men (MSM) (Weeks 1995; Parker, Khan and Aggleton 1998; Cáceres 2002). This phrase is intended to include men who do not regard themselves categorically as 'homosexual' or 'bisexual'.[1] These men may be married, particularly in cultures wherein marriage is strongly promoted by society, and they can be adamant that they are (or find it convenient to consider themselves as) heterosexual.

Growing literature shows that homosexuality exists in traditional African societies (Murray and Roscoe 1998; Niang et al. 2003). The existence of male homosexuality, in particular, has been documented in different parts of Africa (Niang et al. 2003). Sex between males has been reported in prisons in Zambia and Nigeria (Niang et al. 2003) and among migrant factory workers in South Africa (Standing and Kisekka 1989; Niang et al. 2003).[2] Standing and Kisekka (1989) documented the existence of MSM among the Kikuyu in Kenya and the Hausa in Nigeria. The Botswana Ministry of Health reported in 1987 that up to 15% of urban and semi-urban men in Botswana had sexual experience with men (Parker, Khan and Aggleton 1998). Evidence of male-to-male sex has also been explored among Wolof communities, suggesting that the practice is also deeply entrenched in Senegalese society. The prevalence of MSM is higher among Muslim populations (Niang et al. 2003). In contrast, popular and religious discourse reverberates with claims that homosexuality is not an 'African' phenomenon and that homosexuality is 'a foreign disease' (see Epprecht 1998).[3]

Homosexuality in Ethiopia

Hekma argues: 'Every period and culture has produced its own forms of same-sex desires' (1999: 79). Herdt (1997) also maintains that sex between men occurs in almost all cultures and at all times (in Niang et al. 2003). Since the practice is so hidden, one may question if a homosexual community exists in Ethiopia. This is a legitimate question since homosexuality is not widely recognised. Moreover, it is so strongly disapproved of that it is virtually impossible to talk about it openly. It has been the focus of state surveillance and prohibition. Under Article 600 of the Penal Code of 1957, homosexuality is defined as an illegal sexual practice, punishable by imprisonment. Unpublished police annual reports from 1978 to 1987 showed 562 reported cases of homosexuality (Tesfaye 1988). Given that violent and serious crimes are believed severely underreported, Tesfaye argues that this figure may be extremely inaccurate as can be expected for a sexual practice carried out in secret, even between consenting individuals.

The 2005 revised criminal code of Ethiopia still criminalises homosexuality. Article 629 prohibits homosexual acts for both men and women, or 'any other indecent act' with a penalty of 'simple imprisonment'. This penalty may be increased when the offender 'makes a profession of such activities', or exploits a dependency relation in order to exercise influence over the other person. The maximum sentence of ten years' imprisonment can be applied when the offender uses violence, intimidation or coercion, trickery or fraud, or takes unfair advantage of the victim's inability to offer resistance. The maximum sentence can also be applied when the victim is subjected to acts of cruelty or sadism; when the offender transmits a venereal disease although fully aware of being infected with it; when an adult is charged with committing homosexual acts with persons under fifteen years of age; or when distress, shame or despair drives the victim to commit suicide.[4] These legal provisions are rarely enforced, but they give support to institutions such as churches, mosques, or individuals in society to rally against homosexuality.

Research indicates that homosexuality has existed for a long time in different parts of Ethiopia (Murray and Roscoe 1998). My book, *Young Men, Sexuality and HIV/AIDS in an Ethiopian Town* (Tadele 2006) also highlights that homosexuality is present and seems an emerging sexual orientation in a provincial town in Ethiopia.[5] Almost all the street youths involved in the study unanimously remarked that homosexuality is an abhorrent practice and they had never engaged in it. However, they recounted stories of men who had tried to persuade or trick them or their friends into sex. More than half of the schoolchildren who completed a questionnaire appeared familiar with its existence in the town (Tadele 2006).

There is more recent literature that shows the existence of male-to-male sex in Addis Ababa (Hagos 2006; Hagos 2007; Tefera 2007; Ero 2007; Tadele 2007, 2009). With the exception of Hagos's (2007) study, all other studies were conducted in the context of sexual abuse of male children and tangentially revealed the existence of male-to-male sex based on consent. In other words, although these studies had not set out to specifically investigate male-to-male sex, the findings provided evidence of the existence of MSM and male sex work. Hagos's study focuses on 'the possible role of MSM in the epidemiology of HIV/AIDS in Addis Ababa' (2007: 19). He concludes: 'MSM exist and practice in Addis Ababa and a range of factors are said to lead people into such sexual behaviour. As this practice exposes to HIV/AIDS, it must be discussed openly within the context of current efforts to control the HIV pandemic.'

Some magazines, newspapers and blogs have published articles about homosexuality in the last couple of years and brought the existence of homosexual practices among Ethiopians even more forcefully to public attention.[6] There are also blogs such as Meskel Square that discuss homosexuality.[7] Meskel Square has generated highly emotional and sometimes violent rhetoric from both opposing and supporting groups.

This chapter draws from ethnographic data collected from thirty MSM in Addis Ababa, approximately twenty-four in-depth/life-history interviews and one focus group discussion with six participants using the 'snowball' method.[8] Seven were 'elite' informants and the remaining twenty-three worked as 'sex workers'. 'Sex workers' for the purpose of my study refers to those men who claimed that negotiation of sexual intercourse in return for some form of payment constituted their major or main source of income. The term 'elite' refers to those with good economic and social status who claimed not to be involved in sex work. For the purpose of analysing the findings, both sex workers and elites are treated as one group, without necessarily ruling out different sexual experiences.

Although a grounded theory approach to participant observation is difficult in sexuality research, I did my best to participate in social interactions to the extent appropriate.[9] I subscribed to a gay Ethiopian online discussion forum and followed debates, which helped me to frame my research. All informants were 24–33 years old and represented a diversity of ethnic groups and beliefs (Christians-Orthodox, Protestant and Muslims) and life history. The data collection took place between July 2006 and June 2007.

The following sections deal with findings obtained from the fieldwork and all names mentioned in the text are pseudonyms. I refrain from mentioning age and other identifying details in order to protect the identity of informants. I describe sexual identity and vocabulary used by MSM and the public, sexual identity and preference, and the worries and concerns of MSM. I have used verbatim narratives primarily to substantiate my arguments or the claims of informants. I do not reflect on many of the narratives presented in the text in order to allow the readers to generate their own meanings from these texts.

Identity and idiom

Exploring metaphors and idioms that influence thinking about desire and sexuality is a basic element of sociological/anthropological studies of this kind. As Elliston notes:

Such attention to culturally specific metaphors and images about sexuality and eroticism provide crucial insights into the variety of meanings that structure desire and sexuality cross-culturally . . . such images and metaphors could provide the ethnographic detail needed to flesh out the locations and meanings of sexuality and eroticism in different societies (1995: 861).

The words used to name homosexual acts, such as gay or lesbian, predominantly come from the West. In order to conceal their homosexual relationships from the public or heterosexual majority, MSM in Addis Ababa have invented secret idioms and metaphors. They refer to themselves as *Zega*, literally 'citizen', an inclusive term regardless of age and other attributes. Birhanu (an elite informant) put it this way:

In our own lingo, we call ourselves *Zega* irrespective of your preferences, even if you are the active or the passive, you are referred to as a *Zega*. You may be called *wechi* [bottom] or *awchi* [active], and some times you might hear some guys addressing one another as *anchi* [she].

In most cases nicknames and idioms carry a meaningful underlying message. I tried to find out something about the origin and the meaning of *Zega* and other words used by Ethiopian MSM. I asked all my informants carefully why they refer themselves as *Zega*, but failed to generate a satisfactory explanation. One of my elite informants gave two presumptive explanations. First, he argued that the word 'folks' in American English must have been adopted as folk is one possible translation of *Zega* in Amharic (the national language of Ethiopia). Secondly, he thought it might be related to Queer Nation – a gay movement to celebrate gayness, inclusive of gay men, lesbians, bisexuals and transexuals. '*Zega* means we are queer nation, the people from the nation of queer. It means that identifying queerness as second nationality.' Viewed from this perspective, *Zega* has to do with identity concerns and the struggle for respect as citizens, even though their sexuality is different from the mainstream.

Another informant (a sex worker) said that *Zega* is a code name to show that they are not from anywhere else, but are fellow Ethiopians, and they use it to refer to each other without drawing too much attention. He continued: 'It is our code, you know, same as computer codes and the like'. Addressing one another as *Zega* in this case indicates familiarity between the speaker and listener. The term is not only used as a strategy of concealment from the wider society but is also a gesture of belonging and solidarity.

Thus it seems that the word *Zega* is used as a general political statement with layered meanings. It conveys citizenship in narrow sense of identifying like-minded individuals as belonging to a group, subtly conveys that homosexuals are also citizens of Ethiopia and yet is necessarily a code to conceal their sexual disposition in view of the the discrimination they face.

None of the participants used the Amharic words for homosexuality, *Gibre Sodom* (sodomy) or homosexuals, *Gibre Sodomawian*.[10] All the participants expressed a striking sensitivity to the derogatory colloquial word for a homosexual, *bushti*. When asked how he referred to himself, Dawit (a sex worker) instantly reacted that he was a *Zega*. He noted that there were unpleasant words that other people used. When asked which, he replied:

> *Bushti*, if I must say the word. It is just that I hate the word. *Duriyewoch* [hoodlums] call us that most of the time when they want to shame us in front of other people. The very sound of the word disgusts me, we never use it amongst ourselves, and we call each other *Zega*.

Amongst sex workers, there were English and Amharic slang terms used to describe the nature of their activities. 'Businessmen' or sometimes 'bar ladies' were common terms, while those who claimed not to be involved in commercial sex work described those who were as *jerari* or *jerariwoch* (cruising or cruisers). When asked what it means, they said it refers to those who mooch sleeplessly. The term *gomawoch* (tyres) was also used to describe sex workers in reference to the way 'they roll the whole night like the tyres of vehicles'.

Gendered terminology was common and similar to homosexual discourse in other societies (Reid 2007). Participants frequently addressed or referred to individuals as 'she' [*anchi*]. Mikiyas (a sex worker), however, noted that they make a distinction when addressing an 'active' or 'passive' partner in anal intercourse. If the individual plays an insertive role, he is a 'man'. If the individual plays receptive role he is a 'woman' and is addressed as such. In their interpretive framework, those who enjoy being penetrated are structurally equivalent to women. Mikiyas explained the protocol:

> There are like two or three guys I know who are *awchiwoch* [active] and don't like being called *anchi* [she]. They want to be called *ante* [he] and they will be offended if you call them *anchi* and we know this and we call them *ante*. But other than those, I think the rest of us actually like being called *anchi*.
> [How about you, do you like being called that?]
> Yes I do, they call me *anchi* and I call them *anchi*, and we are all happy about it. It is very pleasing, you know.

There were also variable categorisations of general identity. All but two participants said that they consider themselves to be 'gays', using the English word to express themselves.[11] Some who identified themselves as gay also disclosed that they go out with both men and women. Ayele (an elite informant) noted that about 20% of the MSM he knew claim that they are 'pure' gays – they never sleep with women – but the vast majority have some sexual interaction with women. He put in the following words:

> I would say almost all gays whom I know would like to marry and have children in the future. They don't want to stay like this for the rest of their lives. I don't think they will have difficulty to do it as many of them have already girlfriends. Those you interviewed are not the only ones who would like to start [fresh in the] straight world and definitely the majority think that way.

Nonetheless, only one participant, Birhanu, a high-school teacher, identified himself as a heterosexual though he dated men and women. When asked his identity, his reaction was: 'Oh, heterosexual! I think I belong to heterosexual, because a homosexual is someone who never goes beyond same sex [partners]. But I sometimes go beyond that [into heterosexual relations]. So I guess I am more into the heterosexual category than the others.'

Birhanu's consideration of his sexual identity reflects a known phenomenon of claiming a heterosexual identity because it is 'naturalized, normalized and hegemonic' (Flood 2003: 355) and is a clear indicator of the variable criteria that MSM use. For instance, in South Africa, insertive men consider themselves straight, whereas in Brazil only those who penetrate regard themselves as homosexuals (see Reid 2007; Kulick 1997).

Sexual practices and preferences
Sexuality is socially and culturally constructed and people often express different preferences and attitudes with regard to sexual practices: masturbation, anal/oral sex, different sexual positions, erotica and techniques.[12] Tamene (a sex worker) described different sexual positions as follows:

> There is *tebenja bangete* [the rifle around my neck], Argaw Bedaso [the name of a singer from Gurage ethnic group] and *qitel leqema* [collecting leaves]. *Tebenja bangete* is like when the *wechi* [receptive] opens up her legs and puts both legs on the man's shoulder, and the man will creep in from below and do his thing. Argaw Bedaso is when she sits on top and they both sway up and down. *Qitel leqema* is a position whereby the bottom kneels down facing the bed and the top comes and penetrates from behind [he describes action through gestures]. But most of the time, if he is the *awechi* [insertive] and loves the *wechi* [receptive] or if she is his wife, he will have to either suck, lick or masturbate her with his hands so that she can be satisfied. But there is no cuddling among us; we are disgusted by each

other's sight once we have both been satisfied, so we don't even want to be close to one another. But then when we have the urge again, we turn into love birds. And once we both ejaculate, it is back to the same thing all over again. That is just the way it is with us. There are just too many positions and ways. That is why our kind of sex is preferable to that between a man and a woman. I think that is why men prefer us [to girls]. Ours is sweet.

Yosef (a sex worker) maintained that they engage in many kinds of sexual positions, but he distinguished sex for money and for love in the following words:

There is a difference between the sex you do for money and for love. Like when you are paid, you will have to be like what he wants you, he might want you standing up, crouching or bending or lying back, or he might want to do your armpit or ear and so on. And since he is paying, you will have to comply until he is satisfied [*iskeshena*]. Once he has ejaculated, you leave him to his sleep. But when you do it with your lover, you do it with passion and you kiss and stuff. I personally prefer *qitel leqema*.

Abebe (an elite informant) argued that he preferred 'normal' sex, by which he meant lying side by side, adding that he does not much like kissing: 'I haven't done it yet, I haven't. I have never sucked either. But I do have normal sex. I don't like kissing at all; I have only kissed once with the first man I had sex with. I never did it again.'

Within the framework of the top/bottom or active/passive dichotomy in homosexual relationships, I asked all of my informants what they like most. Many stated that they preferred being in the 'top' position but that much depended on the type of relationship and level of intimacy. Sex workers stated that they conformed to the desires of their clients and so would adopt either position though they usually adopted a receptive role during sex because they were being paid to provide a service. Nonetheless, sex workers also stated that they preferred to adopt a receptive role when they wanted to satisfy a person they loved very much. Jemal, a sex worker, explained the issue in the following way:

I practise both. Sometimes if I get someone very good-looking, lovable or someone masculine and dominantly brave, I will let him to penetrate me. But nowadays, I don't make such choices so long as I am paid. If he likes to let you in, you will penetrate him or if your client wants to penetrate you, you will let him in . . . I am currently more inclined to practising the penetration myself. But if my clients are handsome or charming or if they are masculine and well built I enjoy very much receptive role.

Ambivalence, distress and worry: Everyday challenges

I had the feeling even when I was in elementary school, even when I played with my friends back then I was attracted to handsome guys. I didn't give much attention to girls. Later as I grew up, like when I was Grade 7 or 8, I started being attracted towards boys more and more and I was slightly worried by this. I was beginning to ask why I was like that. And all my friends were straight. When I started high school I had this friend, he was straight but we spent a lot of time together. And girls used to approach me for a relationship but I was more in love with him and didn't want a girl. I loved him as a lover could, I thought of him as a lover. But all he knew was that we were good friends. We used to shower together, and we used to do all sorts of things that children do. This went on for about four or five years. But after that he got a girlfriend and introduced me to her. He also told me I should get a girlfriend as well. And I felt like I was very different from people because I didn't know much about it [being gay] back then. I mean I heard about it only at church and that was it. Like in teachings in the church they told us that it was a mortal sin. So I felt different and I was wondering how it was possible to be like this or to happen to me. We had an Internet connection at home, as luck would have it, and I started searching about 'gay' and I read quite a lot about it. I didn't tell anyone about my feeling. I just started searching the Internet and I read quite a lot. I used to take a lot of care so that no one knew what I was reading. I used to delete the browsing history from the computer and all. But I was very worried, so worried that I even went to holy water [*tsebel*] to four or five of the well-known churches. I just prayed by myself, I asked God to help me get out of this thing or if not to give me some one who had the same feelings so that I could at least have some one to talk to and get a relief. So I went on like that for a while. But as I read more and more about it, I came to know that in some countries in Europe, such people could even get married and that there was nothing odd about such a life. And I asked God to correct me but that didn't work and I have accepted that. I don't even consider it as a sin now. It is some-thing inside me and I can't live the rest of my life hiding it.

The above story from an interview with Eyasu, a college graduate, was not atypical. Most of my informants expressed similar concerns and fears when they initially perceived their sexual orientation and it is a common theme in emails on the Ethiopian gay forum. Dagmawi (a sex worker) echoed the same frustration and anxiety when he realised he was attracted to men:

I had been worried too much as I was a devoted Christian. It is regarded as a sin if you are Christian and gay. So, it is not the right thing to do. But, it is something what you are . . . it was from inside. But it was difficult to accept it.

However, he did not have enough words to express his excitement about when he met his first partner:

It was fascinating. It was like a dream to me. I was saying to myself, 'Is there really such a thing? Is this real?' Because I thought I was the only one of my kind that was left. And after I met him, I was thinking we were the only two.

Few informants claimed to have fully overcome their fears of being gay in Ethiopia. For example, Feye asserted:

> I mean it used to worry me a lot, but not now. Because now, I know that I am not alone, I know that there are other people like me and I know where I can find them. I know that there are [plenty] of people in this country who have the same feelings/ desire as me and I know who they are and where I can find them. So I am not worried about that anymore.

Only one participant Ayele (an elite informant) claimed never to have felt 'alone':

> When you see a normal comedy film, you see a gay couple. Then, you start thinking you are not the only one. Many people think they are alone in this city until they find out that there are also others. My worry was how to get the likes of me. Then I found out that there are supportive social groups like gay Ethiopians' Yahoo groups from the Internet. At that time, unfortunately, 90% of the members were foreigners or Ethiopian diaspora. The membership expanded to Ethiopia later. Of course there were problems that made me frustrated. I distanced myself from my friends. I socialised, but have a limit when it came to personal things.

In dominantly heterosexual society where homosexuality is rarely talked about, it is reasonable to assume that those men who find themselves attracted to men should think of themselves as 'the only pebble in the beach'.

Circumventing policed and unconventional sexuality

Living with homophobic families, friends and neighbours was cited as a major challenge by all of my informants. All stated that they had to hide their sexuality. This challenge was acute for those involved in 'business' because they needed to put on make-up and 'feminine' clothing to attract clients. Some informants mentioned that they used their friends' houses to put on make-up and to remove it before returning home. When asked whether any of their family, friends or neighbours knew or suspected their sexual orientation, some informants responded affirmatively. Dagmawi, for instance, said:

I think they know that I am gay even if they don't want to say it. My mother, my aunt and my grandmother know that I am gay though they never confront me. Sometimes my mother tells me why I apply different cosmetics like 'a whore' for more than twelve hours. Actually, the others have never said to me anything like this. They sometimes tell me sarcastically, especially when I have disagreement with them, that it is getting dusk for me to leave as I always take bath and apply cosmetics during this time. They also ask me where I go after washing and making myself so presentable at that time. To appease their curiosity, I tell them that I go to my friends' house to talk about what is currently happening in Deredawa [his birth place]. But my mother asks me why I should wash myself and put all the cosmetics like prostitutes. She also urges me not to apply those cosmetics as I am already handsome. Due to such comments, I suspect that they already knew I am a homosexual even if they never say it to me. My mother is a follower of Protestant religion that strongly condemns our life [homosexuality]. She wants me to be converted into Protestant. She doesn't tell me to abandon homosexuality directly; instead she advises me that being a Protestant enables me to get rid of my addictions [substance abuse]. I get many calls. Thus, she asks me who they are and I tell her that they are my friends who invite me to attend a wedding ceremony. I don't think that this excuse is very satisfactory [for her]. I think they can conclude that I am gay due to the high number of calls I receive. I have neither a fixed telephone nor a mobile. If I have a mobile, I don't think I can control the flow of calls that I get, which definitely can make my families believe that their assumption is right. That is why I don't want to subscribe to get a mobile. There is a kiosk that has a fixed telephone next to our door [home]. I give its telephone number to my friends and customers to avoid my family's assumption. Unfortunately, it doesn't work. I think they know who I am. I prefer to use neighbour's telephone to mobile. If it is mobile, you don't have any alternative but to go outside in order to answer a call when you are at home. They can even hear your telephone conversation outside the home. But if it is in the shop, you can enter inside the shop and talk to the person if the matter is very important. If the case is not that important, you can identify it. I usually tell my customers when they should call me. I wait a call there in the shop not to be called from home. Sometimes, I stay at home and let them call me.

Bitew (a sex worker) reported being terrified when he was seen by his sister-in-law in public:

There is no one in my family who suspects me, but my sister-in-law saw me once wearing disgustingly and standing in a place where gays frequent. I applied make-up and mascara like a woman. I was also wearing a very tight trouser and a kind of clothes that exhibited my tummy when my sister-in-law saw me. Besides, the place where I was seen is frequented by gays. Well, many affluent persons visit the place too. Otherwise, I stay out very late. I always go out from my home giving them a made-up excuse – as a dancer. They do not suspect. You know that there is denial in this country. My families will definitely deny it if I tell them this. So they do not suspect me. But they suspect others. It might be because I am theirs.

Some informants also reported that instead of talking to them and confronting them directly, some families or neighbours strike up a conversation about gays to give 'corrective lessons'. Feye narrated his experience in the following words:

I heard her [his neighbour] when talking with my mother about a naked homosexual pastor, who she said argued with another homosexual over 300 birr that he was supposed to pay for having sex. I left home shockingly when I heard her talking with my mother. I think that they were trying to teach me in order to get me out of this life. They are not frank with me. If they are, I could also tell them honestly that it is my strong feeling, not to interfere with my feeling and I would assure them that I can give up this life whenever I like. I would also tell them that I am the one who live with the sin and die, not they. But, they have never approached to ask me frankly. I have never told them who I am honestly either.

The above examples point to the fact that family members may allude to the sexuality of their children, but do not speak about it directly. In Ethiopia, talking about sexuality with children is a social taboo. As the above statements indicate, MSM use various strategies to conceal their sexual identities and activities. Mikiyas said: 'I have many girlfriends who are girls. It might help me as a cover. Since many girls call home, my father believes that one of them is my girlfriend [lover]. Because of this he doesn't suspect much.' And Jemal talked about how he has to veil his identity:

In fact some of them have accepted that I was a waiter and all the other lies I told them, even though some others are not convinced and usually suspect me as a gay. I usually get startled [shiver] whenever I see them. They do not have good impression towards me. If they knew for sure what I was doing or if I am caught red-handed, I am very certain they would harm or do something bad to me.

An associated fear was being exposed as a result of meeting and socialising openly with gays from the West. Beqalu (a sex worker) narrated his fear in the following terms:

And we have come across scary *ferenjis* [foreigners] at times, you know with their noses pierced and stuff. And I refuse to go out with those types because people would be suspicious if they see you with them out on the streets and I don't want people to know that I do that kind of stuff. We *habeshoch* [Ethiopians] are a long way from that you know. So I ask them if we can just chill inside the house, but they usually want to go out and have fun. But I won't be okay with that and I would leave. You know, I am in this life and that I can't help, but I don't want to put my family to shame by being seen with such people and giving people reason to be suspicious.

An interview with a 'gay foreigner' confirmed Beqalu's fears, as he mentioned that homosexuality is commonly thought to be a practice of 'foreigners' and 'white' people in the country. An underlying feature in these stories was informants' concerns about bringing 'shame' to their families and the difficulties of trying to prevent that happening. As Tamene stated:

I usually do a lot of things at home, like washing clothes and stuff. I don't feel like someone else would wash my clothes as clean as I could. My mom is a bit frail and I often clean the house and make the beds and stuff even when there are girls who can do such things. I want to keep the house tidy and clean. They call me 'Hellen' at home; they said I wasn't a guy [laughs].

However, participants also stated that widespread denial of the existence of homosexuality amongst Ethiopians also served MSM to maintain the fiction. The first thing that comes to parents' minds when their sons spent a lot of the time outside the home is that they are dating girls and they usually warn them about HIV/AIDS. A couple of informants told me that their parents had heard stories about their sexual disposition but refused to acknowledge them as truthful, a common phenomenon elsewhere (Savin-Williams and Dube 1998).

Ethio (an elite informant), for instance, said that he was interrupted by a phone call while writing an email to his gay friend. While he was talking on the phone, his father saw the email and asked what he was writing about. Ethio felt that his his father knew the implication of the email but refused to believe that his son was a homosexual.

The experiences cited above illustrate the code of *Zega* in practice. MSM have created deceptive ways of expressing their sexuality, although they go to great lengths to keep it hidden in a homophobic society. These are tactical manoeuvres in the sense that Shiu-Ki eloquently explains: 'Tactics are ways of making use of the "already-made" cultural system to achieve own desires by introducing alternative meanings to the dominant cultural system. Tactics are an art of the weak or, in Foucault's (1977) terminology, a "technology of the self", or Scott's (1985) idea of "infrapolitics"' (2004: 8).

However, it is a fraught existence. My informants have managed to sustain close familial ties and relationships but in the long run, in the absence of any support or approval at home, their attempts to conceal their sexuality threaten to distance them from their families. There is the potential of breaking away from an intolerant family, friends or neighbourhood, constructing a new environment in which their sexuality can be expressed and so gradually become integrated into a homosexual environment where it is easier for them to reconcile their desire for men. For the moment, anticipating the fact they would be labelled as bad, wrong, unnatural and abnormal left most with uncertainty, resentment, ambivalence, worry and discomfort (see Tadele 2011).

Stigma, harassment and violence

In view of the stigma against homosexuality in Ethiopia, I asked informants – particularly those involved in sex work – to recount their experiences of stigma, harassment and violence. When they were asked about what they hate in this life, they are all afraid of being called *bushti*. Some sex workers argued against the double standard that prevails, where insults and harassment are directed at sex workers and exclude clients. Gudina expressed his rage in the following words:

They throw stones and insult us should we stand in a group. If they see us in a group at the same place and all times, they would do anything to get rid of us from that place labeling us *bushtiwoch* [plural]. For instance, National Theatre is well known as our concentration area, so are Piassa and Bole area. If we stand, walk or pace around these places in a group, they insult us knowing that we are gays and waiting for business. They see many authorities, celebrities and rich people picking us. They have never said anything to these people as they have power and money. I don't know why they insult us instead. I wish they wouldn't call us names. Nobody touches those gays who have power and money.

Bitew also mentioned the verbal abuse as well as physical intimidation:

No one would let you use the path unless you move from one car to another or from one car to the bar to entertain yourself. They call you names such as *bushti*. I am so afraid of such insults that I can't wear clothes and make-up, which I am supposed to do in order to attract my customers. As a result, the income that I get from this business is drastically plummeting . . . I told you that they easily identify us by our wearing style and the places where we hang out. Of course, straights also wear 'vale' trousers, but they could identify us as gays easily as our walking is unique. Then, they call us names. Sometimes they beat and spit at you. They accuse us of tarnishing Ethiopia when we asked them why they were doing that to us. Even in a hotel, they insult you while you are dancing. They splash beer on you and beat you with [beer] bottles sometimes.

Other commercial sex workers cited physical abuse they had experienced. Dawit explained:

There are hooligans who force us to give them money during night time. Some know us and tell to others that we are gays.

Then, they beat us up and take our money. Sometimes, we go to a hotel or take a hooligan to our home [inadvertently] as a client, then he beats us up and robs our property. They wait for you in an unsafe place. They even humiliate you in front of people. They express their hatred. They also take your mobile, gold and money that you have at that time. If you don't have, they tell you to bring some another time.

Dawit attributed such violence to the illegality of homosexuality and the attackers counting that their victims would not take the cases to court:

The fear contributes a lot in that. I mean there are guys who get beaten nearly to death and robbed. If some thug [*duriye*] discovers that you are gay, he would wait for you at some dark street corner and start calling you *bushti* and take a swing at you and rob you if he can. But if it became legal, no one would be able to touch you. That is what I think.

Personal experiences of phycial violence were harrowing, as Dawit's testimony reveals:

There was this one time we were going together with this guy I met and made a deal with. We were going to rent a room for the night when a bunch of guys came from nowhere and started calling us *bushtiwoch* and all. I guess they knew the guy I was with was gay. We tried to run away but we didn't get far, they caught up with us and they started beating us up. I told them they could take everything I have, and they slapped me around a bit and they took my mobile phone and all my money and didn't hurt me much. But they gave the guy I was with a good beating and they also took his mobile and his money. I went to the police to report that I have been robbed later on but they didn't seem to care. They asked me to bring a witness. There were a few hookers who saw what happened but they didn't want to be witnesses, they said they haven't seen a thing. I was furious for a while; it was like there was no law in the country. But after a while, I had to let go, there was nothing I could do about it. And I was at least thankful that they didn't hurt me much.

Zeberga (a sex worker) recounted a being raped by a gang:

There were these guys around the Hilton, they used to see me hanging out around there a lot. And this one time, I came across them past midnight, around 1.00 a.m., and I was a bit drunk. I was with some *ferenjis* at the Hilton the whole evening but I didn't want to have sex that day and I said goodbye and went out to go home. But I couldn't find a taxi and these guys came over to me and said hi. I said hi as well and asked them if they would like a few drinks, they said okay and we went to this pub together. They ordered some draught [beer] and I paid for the drinks and told them I would pay for the drinks if they wanted to order more but I can't stay with them that I had to go home. But they would have none of that. They said they wanted to have sex with me. They took me to this back alley and beat me up and had sex with me. All three of them. Like one would have me suck him while the other was fucking me from behind. I thought of shouting for help but it was a very quiet place and I didn't think anyone would come for help [to my rescue]. I tried to struggle with them a bit and tried to scream but they started beating me up so badly. So I thought it would be better to have sex with them than being beaten to death. They just forced me to have sex with them, they were saying things like '*ante ferenj iyasgeba sibedah igna isti zur ferenj yayewin igna mayet anchilim*' [every *ferenji* gets to fuck you, how come we can't see what you show the *ferenjis*, so bend over]. And I was happy to comply . . . I mean they had torn my shirt to pieces and they were trying to get my trousers off. I tried to hold on to my trousers as much as I could but in the end, I couldn't stand up to all three of them. It was in this open space beyond the Hilton and it was dark and I had no chance [of fighting them off]. So I had to comply, I had no other choice. And once they were through with me, they warned me not to say a single word to anyone about what just happened or they would kill me.

And, on another occasion:

The police took me and said they have received information that I engage in homosexual sex and I said that it is indeed correct and I do but I have never raped anyone or done it without the consent of a partner. And the commander of the police station was furious when he heard me saying that. He screamed, 'Are you telling me that you are a *bushti?*' and hit me on my forehead with the butt of his pistol. And I objected that there is no reason why he should hit me, that I haven't forced any one to have sex with me, that all I have done is satisfy my feeling with someone else who had the same feelings [*yewiste simet new beqa yenekahut yasgededkut sew yelem*]. They held me for about one month and then they took me to court . . .

Ayele (an elite informant) also narrated a story of a gay person who was detained and went through a horrible experience. The police caught two men having oral sex near the St George Church in Addis Ababa. The police arrested, tied and beat them and told them that they would be released if they told the truth and gave out other gays' names. A person whose name was given to the police in this way was arrested in Piassa, a locality in Addis Ababa:

The police took him along with others and locked him without any evidence. There were around twenty people who were locked up. All of them denied the allegation. But, they were beaten extremely. He had been in prison for three months along with twenty alleged homosexuals without being taken to the court. He was bailed out at last. Even after being released, he was abused by the police. The police threatened his mother that they would arrest him again unless she bribed them some money and his family suffered a lot. Finally, they were able to send him to England. I even asked him why he doesn't write it and share it to the Yahoo groups. He told me that it is a long story and he would like to write a book about it.

Ayele continued and said:

Another incidence is that my straight classmate happened to be at a place where marijuana was available. He had nothing with this drug. Unfortunately, the police overran the place and arrested him together with others. He was released after being detained for five days at Federal Police Station. My classmate told me what he saw in that police station and narrated that there was a gay who received unspeakable maltreatment not only from police officers but also other detainees because he is gay. He was forced to sleep next to a latrine. They called the gay by the name of Aster [a feminine name].

These experiences suggest that there is sporadic, extra-judicial enforcement of the law against homosexuality in Addis Ababa, exacerbated by the notoriously harsh conditions of Ethiopia's prisons. The police officers I interviewed affirmed the tenor of my informants' stories.[13]

Amidst these experiences, there were also reports of how MSM employ various tactics to evade abuse, which in part rely on the conservative social values that prevail in Ethiopia. Jemal recounted the following experience:

I have been once caught by a policeman and I was very melancholic and told him all my problems. He felt very sad about my story and advised me to pray and remember always God so that I can give up this sexuality and set myself free very sooner. If I am caught I would admit that I am gay politely and with regret and tell the policemen all the stories and that I am not happy at all in this gay life, just like what I am telling you right now. And I am very persuasive and they usually let me go after giving me some pieces of advice. If some guys deny that they are gays and try to lie to the policemen, they [the police] will hate them for being cheaters and will beat them, tear their clothes and inflict on them all sorts of harassments.

Self-stigma

Self-stigma, in the sense of internalised homophobic attitudes, was evident in the vast majority of my informants. For example, when I asked Dawit to tell me what troubles him and what pleases him in his life, he said:

> I want to abandon this life and start a new one. The mere thought of this [giving up homosexuality] makes me happy . . . You become paranoid when you become gay. You think everyone knows your sexuality. It is not only because of your walking or wearing style. I get also nervous when a person stares at me thinking that he knows that I am gay. I make myself so worried although the person doesn't have any idea about my sexuality.

In line with Goffman's (1963) discussion of stigma, Dawit's interactions with society are cautious. He feels that whoever looks at him knows his sexuality and will not accept him on equal ground. It appears that his relationships with other people are always tempered with a lot of fear, insecurity and vigilance. Statements such as 'I don't want my family to find out about my sexuality. I don't want them to feel sorry' also show how he is preoccupied with family loyalty. He implied that, to his family, being gay is evil and perverted and he could not stand the idea of them knowing that one of their own is gay.

On a later occasion, I met Dawit to find that he had grown a beard to prevent being identified as gay and to appear more 'manly'. However, he struggled to reconcile the contradictions of this tactic in his response to my questioning whether the beard had affected his sex work, in terms of attracting clients:

> The clients like you when you keep yourself and your hygiene. They like you when you look beautiful and dressed well. They don't like you when you look messed up. But I do not have a choice but to grow beard to avoid public scrutiny. When you keep yourself presentable and dressed well, the clients respect you. Even those who have known you for a long time, like you when they see you smartly dressed and changed well. Sometimes it is good to act like a man. But for the business, it is preferable to be well dressed and presentable like a woman, which sometimes turned out to be disgusting. When you feel not happy acting and wearing like a woman, it is good to be a man.

Suicide and attempted suicide are known to be associated with the emotional turmoil over sexual disposition and societal prejudices surrounding same-sex relationships (Hillier and Harrison 2004: 80). There are no accurate statistics of suicide rates in Ethiopia and I did not investigate the issue. However, Ayele (an elite informant) reported:

> I know many young people who wanted to commit suicide due to extreme pressure and failure of accepting that they are gays. Even those who are educated express their disgust towards homosexuals. The boy I told you about, who tried to commit suicide, is from a well-educated family. His mother is a well-educated woman and got her education abroad. She is now working for a big NGO [non-governmental organisation]. She expresses her extreme disgust for homosexuality in her routine chat at home. She doesn't have any idea that her son is a gay. There is no doubt that she would kill him should she finds out.

Depression and self-stigmatisation was common amongst my informants and expressed in other ways. For example, almost all informants expressed their desire to migrate to other countries, notably to Western Europe or North America. Zeberga was adamant:

> Nothing would make me happier . . . so that I can live and be as I wish. It is not like that here, I am always thinking about what others might think [if they knew I was gay], you know, here you always feel like someone is watching you. So you are never free to be as you please. And besides, there would be opportunities abroad for you to improve yourself and be someone. I wouldn't get such opportunities if I stay here.

Likewise many were equivocal about their future and the health risks in the context of HIV/AIDS. Feye commented:

> If I am going to live in this country, I have a girl that I consider mine and I think when the time comes, we will get married. But if I can go abroad and meet some guy that I can love and make mine, I would rather go on living this life there [continue living as gay]. But as long as I am in this country, I wouldn't think of it.

With regard to the sexual health risks, my information supported a common argument in the research literature of a possible association between increased rates of unprotected anal intercourse and emotional depression (Dudley et al. 2004). There was evidence of misconceptions amongst my informants about the risks taken by MSM. For example, Zeberga stated: 'I think it is more risky to have sex with a woman. From what I know [have heard] I think the contact there is a lot more risky. I don't think it is transmitted that much through unprotected male-to-male sex.'

I frequently heard statements in this vein from the sex workers and also from a couple of elite informants (see Tadele 2010). While these misconceptions can be attributed to the lack of public health messages directed at MSM in Ethiopia, there are also subliminal factors that cannot be ignored. For instance, there are codes of behaviour, indeed rituals, amongst the sex workers that encourage not using condoms, which are linked to belief in spirits and spirit possession (see Tadele 2010).

Conclusion

My study on MSM in Addis Ababa revealed the desperation of 'gays' in the country, which they aptly expressed in their use of the word *Zega* (citizen) to describe themselves as a particular sub-population in Ethiopia. They clearly were not regarded as citizens in the formal sense, in view of the prejudice and abuse they faced from the broader society and the illegality of homosexuality. Yet, in using the identity of *Zega*, MSM in Addis Ababa were conveying both resistance to the abuse and a yearning to be acknowledged as citizens. Citizenship includes sexual disposition as a criterion for defining membership of society; MSM are not 'citizens' because heterosexuality is upheld in Ethiopian society as both an ideal and practice of being a citizen. This is not peculiar to Ethiopia (Stychin 2003) but there is resistance to this prejudice, openly conveyed in the motto, 'Ethiopian by birth, Gay by nature and PROUD by choice' on the Ethiopian 'gay' website.[14] Though this motto seems to draw on international and probably North American networks through the choice of words and language, there is also an intimation of an appeal to the Ethiopian public that being 'gay' is not only the practice of 'foreigners' (*ferenjis*).

Contrary to the widespread public denial about homosexuality in Ethiopian society, my research shows that male-to-male sexual relationships are an entrenched part of the social fabric and there is a flourishing underground sex trade. Equally, the prejudice and abuse fostered by the state cannot be understated. These findings warrant attention in Ethiopia for the prevention of HIV/AIDS among this group and the general public.

Sexuality has increasingly come to be viewed as a positive lifelong activity and fundamental to being human. Hence sexual health and rights have also come to be viewed as an integral part of a human rights framework. The concept of sexual health 'includes healthy sexual development, equitable and responsible relationships and sexual fulfilment, freedom from illness, disease, disability, violence and other harmful practices related to sexuality'.[15] The concept of sexual rights includes

> the ability to maintain personal preferences regarding whatever ways one exercises his or her sexual feeling in order to attain a high standard of sexuality, including the pursuit of a satisfying and safe and pleasurable sexual life, and the decision to enter into sexual relations and marriage wilfully. Within this premise, each man and woman determines what is best for him or her regarding sexual expression (Ojo 2007: 144).

This study therefore contends that there is a pressing need to open up space for discussions about different sexual practices and forms of relationships that take place in Ethiopa. I believe that we must examine the issue before it is too late to reverse the damage that HIV/AIDS may cause in the MSM community and the public at large. There is a need for debate on the reality of the situation instead of a moralising discourse that denies male-to-male sex. We must overcome the denial in the face of knowledge that can prevent morbidity and mortality by HIV/AIDS and improve the lives of many in other ways. Some of my informants admitted that they also had sex with women, thereby indicating the potential of HIV transmission in society driven by risky sex between men. There is an urgent need to accept that MSM exist and that risky sexual practices are more common than Ethiopians care to acknowledge. Ethiopians cannot talk about the problem of HIV/AIDS and yet ignore some obvious channels for the transmission of the virus and approaches to protect and support those at risk.

Notes
1. The term, MSM is further intended to include all types of male-to-male sexual relationships that share similar levels of HIV risk as gay relationships (Cáceres 2002).

2. The findings from prisons indicate that although most same-sex behavior is practised by choice, institutions such as prisons, military and other similar situations in which men are obliged to spend long periods in all-male company create conditions that promote same sex relationships.

3. According to the International Gay and Lesbian Association, homosexuality is outlawed in 38 African countries and legal (or not mentioned in the statute books) in at least 13 countries (see http://news.bbc.co.uk/2/hi/africa/7266646.stm).

4. Proclamation No. 414/2004 of 2005: The Criminal Code of the Federal Democratic Republic of Ethiopia: Articles 629-33.

5. The book focuses on young people's perceptions of sex, love, marriage and HIV/AIDS in the context of poverty and ongoing HIV/AIDS intervention programmes. It also discusses young people's perceptions of homosexuality very briefly.

6. See *Mezenagna* (Entertainment) Amharic newspaper (2 April 2005; *Megabit* 25, 1999 Ethiopian Calendar); *Zemen Magazine* (24 January 2007) and *My Fashion* magazine (May 2006).

7. See www.meskelsquare.com/archives/2005/04/holding_hands.html.

8. Snowball sampling involves using those informants contacted in one way or another to recruit their associates and friends. It is also refered as respondent-driven sampling.

9. This is more complicated since I am a straight married man studying MSM and I might have misrepresented some of the subtle meanings and symbolism in the narratives of the MSM who participated in the study. Further, as a university teacher relatively older than most informants, I do not share many membership attributes with them. Being an insider and on equal footing, however, does not guarantee the production of valid and reliable data. I would also like to state that the small sample size, dominated by sex workers, raises concerns about representation of MSM from different walks of life.

10. *Gibre Sodom* is Ge'ez (Ethiopic language mainly used in the liturgy of the Ethiopian Orthodox Tewahedo Church) word that translates literarally as the 'work or practice of sodomites'.

11. Mamush (an elite informant) claimed that he dated women as well but he said that he is confused about his sexual identity and does not identify himself as gay.

12. There is also a variety of terminology to describe different practices; for example, oral sex or felatio is referred to as 'singing', in reference to the resemblance of a man's penis to a stage microphone and the act of holding it.

13. In 2007, I conducted consultancy research on sexual abuse against male street children (see Tadele 2007, 2009). This research gave me an opportunity to conduct interviews with members of the criminal justice system and other key informants working for government and non-governmental, child-focused

organisations and I broached a number of issues related to homosexuality in the context of this research. Otherwise, since it is illegal it would have been difficult to present myself as a researcher on homosexuality.

14. See www.gayethiopians.com/Home.htm.
15. See www.icw.org/files/SRHR-ICW%20fact%20sheet-06.doc.

References

Cáceres, C. 2002. 'HIV among Gay and Other Men Who Have Sex with Men in Latin America and the Caribbean: A Hidden Epidemic?' *AIDS* 16(3): S23–S33.

Dudley, M.G., S.S. Rostosky, B.A. Korfhage and R.S. Zimmerman. 2004. 'Correlates of High-Risk Sexual Behavior among Young Men Who Have Sex with Men'. *AIDS Education and Prevention* 16(4): 328–40.

Elliston, D. 1995. 'Erotic Anthroplogy: "Ritualized Homosexuality" in Melenesia and Beyond'. *American Anthropologist* 22(4): 848–67.

Epprecht, M. 1998. 'The "Unsaying" of Indigenous Homosexualities in Zimbabwe: Mapping a Blind Spot in an African Masculinity'. *Journal of Southern African Studies* 24(4): 631–51.

Ero, D. 2007. 'Sexual Abuse of Male Children in Addis Ababa'. M.A. thesis. Addis Ababa: School of Social Work, Addis Ababa University.

Flood, M. 2003. 'Lust, Trust and Latex: Why Young Heterosexual Men Do Not Use Condoms'. *Culture, Health & Sexuality* 5(4): 353–69.

Goffman, E. 1963. *Stigma: Notes on the Management of Spoiled Identity*. New Jersey: Prentice-Hall.

Hagos, B. 2006. *Sexual Abuse and Exploitation of Male Children in Addis Ababa*. Addis Ababa: Save the Children (Denmark) and Bright for Children Voluntary Association.

Hagos, S. 2007. 'Assessment of HIV/AIDS Related Risks among Men Having Sex with Men (MSM) in Addis Ababa'. Extracts from EPHA-Sponsored Master's Theses in HIV/AIDS. Ethiopian Public Health Association. Addis Ababa.

Hekma, G. 1999. 'Same-Sex Relations among Men in Europe, 1700–1900'. In F.X. Eder, L.A Hall and G. Hekma (eds). *Sexual Cultures in Europe: Themes in Sexuality*. Manchester: Manchester University Press: 79–103.

Hillier, L. and L. Harrison. 2004. 'Homophobia and the Production of Shame: Young People and Same Sex Attraction'. *Culture, Health & Sexuality* 6(1): 79–94.

Kulick, D. 1997. 'The Gender of Brazilian Transgendered Prostitutes'. *American Anthropologist* 99(3): 574–85.

Murray, S. and W. Roscoe. 1998. *Boy-Wives and Female Husbands: Studies in African Homosexualities*. New York: Palgrave.

Niang, C.I., P. Tapsoba, E. Weiss, M. Diagne, Y. Niang, A.M. Moreau, D. Gomis, A.S. Wade, K. Seck and C. Castle. 2003. ' "It's Raining Stones": Stigma, Violence and HIV Vulnerability among Men Who Have Sex with Men in Dakar, Senegal'. *Culture, Health & Sexuality* 5(6): 499–512.

Ojo, M. 2007. 'Religion and Sexuality: Individuality, Choice and Sexual Rights in Nigerian Christianity'. In E. Maticka-Tyndale, R. Tiemoko and P. Makinwa-Adebusoye (eds). *Human Sexuality in Africa: Beyond Reproduction*. Auckland Park: Fanele: 131–48.

Parker, R., S. Khan and P. Aggleton. 1998. 'Conspicuous by Their Absence? Men Who Have Sex with Men (MSM) in Developing Countries: Implications for HIV Prevention'. *Critical Public Health* 8: 329–46.

Parker, R.G. and J.H. Gagnon (eds). *Conceiving Sexuality: Approaches to Sex Research in a Postmodern World*. New York: Routledge.

Reid, G. 2007. 'How to be a "Real Gay": Emerging Gay Spaces in Small-Town South Africa'. Ph.D. dissertation. Amsterdam: University of Amsterdam.

Savin-Williams, R.C. and E. Dube. 1998. 'Parental Reaction to Their Child's Disclosure of a Gay/Lesbian Identity'. *Family Relations* 47(1): 7–13.

Shiu-Ki, T. 2004. 'Queer at Your Own Risk: Marginality, Community and Hong Kong Gay Male Bodies'. *Sexualities* 7(1): 5–30.

Standing, H. and M.N. Kisekka. 1989. 'Sexual Behavior in Sub-Saharan Africa: A Review and Annotated Bibliography'. Unpublished.

Stychin, C. 2003. *Governing Sexuality: The Changing Politics of Citizenship and Law Reform*. Oxford: HART Publishing.

Tadele, G. 2006. *Young Men, Sexuality and HIV/AIDS in an Ethiopian Town*. Leiden: African Studies Centre.

———. 2007. 'The Situation of Sexual Abuse against Male Street Children in Merkato Area, Addis Ababa'. Consultancy research report sponsored by Forum on Street Children Ethiopia in collaboration with Save the Children, Sweden.

———. 2009. ' "Unrecognized Victims": Sexual Abuse against Male Street Children in Merkato Area, Addis Ababa'. *Ethiopian Journal of Health Development* 23(3): 174–82.

———. 2010. ' "Boundaries of Sexual Safety": Men Who Have Sex with Men (MSM) and HIV/AIDS in Addis Ababa'. *Journal of HIV/AIDS and Social Services* 9(3): 261–80.

———. 2011. 'Heteronormativity and "Troubled" Masculinities among Men Who Have Sex with Men (MSM) in Addis Ababa'. *Culture, Health & Sexuality* 13(4): 457–69.

Tefera, A. 2007. 'Sexual Abuse against Male Children in Addis Ababa'. B.A. thesis. Addis Ababa: Department of Sociology and Social Anthropology, Addis Ababa University.

Tesfaye, A. 1988. 'The Crime Problem and its Correction' (Vol. I). Addis Ababa: Department of Sociology and Social Administration, Addis Ababa University.

Weeks, J. 1995. 'History, Desire and Identities'. In R.G. Parker and J.H. Gagnon (eds). *Conceiving Sexuality: Approaches to Sex Research in a Postmodern World*. New York: Routledge: 34–50.

9

Race and HIV/AIDS in Public Health Discourse in Africa

Ademola J. Ajuwon

Race and ethnicity are persistent, significant themes in public discourse on HIV/AIDS. Surveillance data and public discussion on sexually transmitted infections (STIs) and HIV infection suggest that 'blacks', including those living in sub-Saharan Africa and in the diaspora, are at increased risk of acquiring and spreading HIV. This has indirectly created a public perception that AIDS is a 'black problem'. Yet there are no known biological reasons to explain why racial or ethnic factors alone should alter the risk for STIs or HIV. It is the behaviour of an individual and not the colour of his skin that determines the risk of HIV infection. This chapter provides an overview of how race and ethnicity are ingrained in public discourse on HIV/AIDS and a backdrop to the detailed illustrations that appear in other chapters.

In the early 1980s, HIV was a fatal disease that devastated the lives of affected people, their families and communities. However the introduction of antiretroviral (ARV) therapy in the 1990s changed the profile of HIV from being a death sentence to a manageable disease (Fenton, Johnson and Nicoll 1997). ARVs are now widely available in many countries in Europe and North America but the majority of people who need treatment in sub-Saharan Africa do not have access to ARVs. Reportedly only about 30% of HIV-infected people living in resource-poor settings have access to treatment (UNAIDS/WHO 2008).

Popular and scientific debates on these challenges have highlighted the dissonance in various ways, including questioning the ethics of large-scale HIV vaccine research in Africa (Guenter, Esparza and Macklin 2000), the inequalities in access to ARVs between HIV-infected persons living in resource-poor settings and their counterparts living in wealthy nations (Greenberg et al. 2008), the ethical conduct of HIV/AIDS research in sub-Saharan Africa by scientists from developed countries (Marshall 2005; Lurie and Wolfe 1997) and, most recently, the advocacy of male circumcision (Auvert et al. 2005; Gray et al. 2007; Bailey et al. 2007).

Race and ethnicity are often subliminal in these debates, while scientific studies on the 'impact' of HIV/AIDS regularly make overt references. For instance, in the 1990s, surveillance data on STIs and HIV among different racial groups in selected cities in the United States and United Kingdom suggested that people of African descent were at higher risk of infection (St Louis, Farley and Aral 1996; Lacey et al. 1997).

One effect has been confusion as to *why*, or indeed, *whether* race and ethnicity are pertinent factors in understanding the HIV/AIDS pandemic. On the one hand, race and ethnicity alone are not risk factors for HIV (CDC 2008) and there are no known biological reasons to explain why racial or ethnic factors alone should alter the risk (Fenton, Johnson and Nicoll 1997). Consequently, these concepts should be disavowed as prejudicial constructs that foster discrimination in a context where there is already much discrimination and stigma associated with HIV/AIDS. On the other hand, these concepts help to identify epidemiological patterns and trends of the pandemic.

The current HIV and AIDS situation in Africa

General features of the HIV/AIDS pandemic in Africa are briefly outlined below for, as is indicated later, the variations in epidemiological trends are a source of the confusion and abuse of the concepts of race and ethnicity in public discourses on the disease.

Sub-Saharan Africa is disproportionately affected by the impact of AIDS. Of the 4.3 million new global infections for 2006 alone,

2.8 million or 66% were from sub-Saharan Africa and 2.1 million persons died of AIDS (Greenberg et al. 2008). In addition, approximately 14 million children have been orphaned by the disease so far (UNAIDS 2009). AIDS is now a huge burden on African healthcare systems (Wanyenze et al. 2008), many of which are already overburdened by high levels of many communicable diseases, including malaria, diarrhoea and tuberculosis. The epidemic has spread steadily with a concomitant fall in life expectancy in some African countries. For example, in Nigeria, life expectancy dropped from 53 years in 1990 to 44 years in 2005 (NIBUCAA 2007). In South Africa, life expectancy declined from 59 years in the early 1990s to 45 in the late 1990s (Van Niekerk 2002).

The scale of national epidemics varies considerably across the continent. For example, countries in the southern African region – South Africa, Lesotho, Swaziland, Botswana, Namibia, Zambia and Zimbabwe – have the largest epidemics. The national adult HIV prevalence in each of these countries exceeds 15%. In 2007, this region accounted for almost a third (32%) of all new HIV infections and AIDS-related deaths globally (UNAIDS/WHO 2008). By contrast, none of the countries in West Africa have HIV prevalence rates above 10% (UNAIDS/WHO 2008). However, percentage assessments can be misleading. For instance, the prevalence of 4.4% of adult Nigerians infected with HIV in 2005 (FMOH 2006) was smaller than those of many eastern and southern African countries. But Nigeria's large population means that almost 3.5 million Nigerians were living with HIV in 2005, second in number globally only to South Africa (UNAIDS/WHO 2008). There are also state or provincial variations within countries. For example, in 2005, Benue state in central Nigeria had a prevalence rate of 10% compared to 4.4% for the entire country (FMOH 2006). In South Africa, KwaZulu-Natal province had and continues to have the highest prevalence (16%) whereas the Western Cape has the lowest (6%) (Metam 2008).

The concepts of race and ethnicity
Race refers to a population that shares hereditary and physical features (Landis 1974). The general reference to a population that has particular

features is commonly abbreviated into geographical distinction of three races: African, Caucasian and Asian, with variations over time identifying other races, such as American Indians, Australian aborigines (Bhopal 1997) and terminology (for example, 'black', 'white', 'Mongoloid'). Racialisation refers to the idea that race is a primary, natural and useful means of grouping human beings and to the attribution of distinct behaviours amongst each population (Bhopal 1997). Racialism or racism is the expression of belief in the superiority of some races (Bharat 2003).

Race is a problematic concept because there are no clear boundaries between the designated populations. There is as much physical variation within 'races' as there is between 'races' and there is also as much physical commonality as difference between 'races'. Hence attributions of distinct behaviours and hierarchy are spurious (Landis 1974). To illustrate, common use of skin colour as a distinguishing characteristic (physical phenotype) to define Africans is also prevalent in unrelated populations on the Indian subcontinent, in Australia, New Guinea and elsewhere in the southwest Pacific (O'Neil 2008).

A concept closely related to race is ethnicity. Ethnicity refers to a population that shares ancestral and geographical origins, cultural traditions and languages (Bhopal 1997). Common discourse uses the term 'ethnic groups' to distinguish these populations – for example, the Yoruba, Hausa and Igbo in Nigeria; the Twi and Ewe in Ghana; and the Zulu, Xhosa and Sotho populations in South Africa. Variations in terminology over time are common; for instance, 'tribe', 'culture' and 'nation'. As with the concept of race, ethnicity is frequently imbued with judgement – for example, stereotyping an individual's behaviour as a function of that person's origins or culture.

Likewise, 'minority' has become a common term in modern times. It is used to describe a group that is numerically smaller than other groups within a national population; to refer to cultural, religious or linguistic characteristics that are different from a general 'national' culture; and to indicate either political solidarity on the part of that group in relation to others and the national population or to a disadvantaged status within a larger population (O'Neil 2008). Notably, 'minority' has become a means to draw attention to inequalities and injustices that prevail in particular populations, such as the aboriginal people in Australia, Maoris and Solomon Islanders in New Zealand and Inuit in Canada (UNESCO 2002). In Africa, similar examples abound – for instance, in Nigeria, the Osu caste among the Igbos of southeastern Nigeria are routinely discriminated against and stigmatised.

Race and ethnicity in health science
Race and ethnicity have been used frequently, overtly and subliminally, in popular, scientific and policy explanations of the aetiology and epidemiology of diseases and discussions of disparities in health conditions and outcomes (Fenton, Johnson and Nicoll 1997). For instance, it is now widely publicised that African-Americans in the United States and 'blacks' in England and Wales have higher HIV prevalence rates than other 'races' (Dougan et al. 2004). In South Africa, demographic modelling of HIV prevalence uses the country's long-standing (slightly modified since 1994) categorisation of people into racially defined 'population groups' ('white', 'black', 'Indian', 'Coloured') (Dilraj, Abdool Karim and Pillay 2007). In this case, there is also the practice, in public discourse and in government and scientific documents, of sometimes replacing the category 'black' with the term 'African'.[1] The irony is that such manipulation allows for racially exclusive views of who is or who may be categorised as 'African'.

Similarly, race, along with sex and class, is often used as a marker for demographic surveillance of diseases and to inform public health strategies and policies, prediction of the statistical probability of illness and well-being, and assessments of health-seeking and coping behaviours and accessibility to services (Fenton, Johnson and Nicoll 1997; Bharat 2003). In Canada, surveys suggested that HIV prevalence was highest amongst Inuit people; in Honduras (in 1991) HIV prevalence was six times higher among the Garifuna communities (a minority group) on the Atlantic coast than it was among the general population (UNESCO 2002); in Nigeria, the state of Benue, located in the north central region of the country, was identified as the state with the highest HIV prevalence rate (FMOH 2006).

Inevitably, such use is fraught with confusion and controversy. In South Africa, the persistent perception that HIV/AIDS is a 'black problem' (Dilraj, Abdool Karim and Pillay 2007) confuses and discriminates on at least four grounds. First, it infers that the disease is not a 'problem' (insignificant prevalence rates) amongst the 'white', 'Indian' and 'Coloured' populations, thereby misrepresenting the threat and presence of HIV and AIDS in that country's population. The percentage prevalence rates may indeed be much lower in these categories. Dilraj, Abdool Karim and Pillay (2007), for instance, recorded 1.1% HIV prevalence amongst 'Indians' and 4.4% amongst 'Coloureds', compared to general rates of 24.8% amongst 'blacks'. However, as mentioned earlier, percentages are misleading when absolute numbers of HIV-infected persons are high. Second is the simplistic summation of demographic patterns of HIV infection: estimates of HIV prevalence show highest rates amongst the 'black' population; the majority of the population are 'black'; therefore, that is *the* location (as opposed to other population categories of the country's HIV epidemic). Third, the racial profiling in official and scientific estimates of HIV prevalence in South Africa encourages this perception, in part because qualifications and caveats behind them are usually not considered in public discourse. For example, 'black' South Africans are over-represented in the data from public health service antenatal clinics, which is a primary source for estimating national HIV-prevalence rates. The majority (89.4%) of all pregnant women tested at the antenatal clinics in the country are 'black' South Africans; the majority of 'white' South African women use private health clinics, which are not included in national compilations of the data. Fourth, there are much more precise categories based on socio-economic factors that can be and are used to differentiate levels of risk and prevalence within a national population.

In a related manner, the conclusion of scientific studies that 'black' people suffer lower levels of good health than 'whites', due in part to different genetic traits, generated much debate (Marshall 2005; Greenberg et al. 2008). Similarly, the confusion of racial and ethnic categorisations with social conditions calls into question the conclusions of similar studies, such as African-Americans ('blacks') engaging more frequently than 'white' and 'Hispanic' Americans in 'health-risk' behaviours (for example, alcohol use and sex with multiple partners) (Greenberg et al. 2008).

The problem, the potential for abuse of these representations of patterns and trends in health and disease, is that the structural factors that create situations for high prevalence rates in these populations are seldom given adequate consideration in the research and in the planning of interventions (Springer 1998). In many communities, 'minority' groups are economically and politically disadvantaged compared with other segments of the population. Consequently, there is higher incidence of 'health risk' behaviour within those populations that are reflected in statistical compilations of data (see, for example, Chapters 7 and 10 in this volume). Furthermore, the effects of diseases such as HIV/AIDS can be more devastating amongst poor populations than amongst wealthier populations because the former have limited access to the healthcare system (UNESCO 2002).

An equally fraught issue is the conducting of research on diseases. A classic example of racial discrimination in research was the Tuskegee study on syphilis among 'African-American' men in the United States. In 1932, a prospective study commenced among 300 'African-American' men with syphilis in Macon County, Alabama, to determine the natural history of this disease. These men were not informed of their disease nor were they told that the research would not benefit them. They were deceived into receiving treatment for 'bad blood', the euphemism for syphilis (Dunn and Chadwick 1999). Furthermore, penicillin became available in 1943 and was effective in curing syphilis but the affected men were not informed of the medical advance and were not treated, for the sake of maintaining the 'scientific' integrity of the experiments.

A vast amount of clinical research on HIV/AIDS in Africa includes unethical studies. For example, a controlled trial conducted by Quinn and colleagues (2000) in the Rakai district of Uganda examined the natural history of HIV infection among sero-discordant couples who were not informed about their partners' HIV status. In this decade, there has been growing concern amongst African scholars that Africans are being used as 'guinea pigs'. This is a phrase frequently used in discussions at conferences in Africa. The polemic subsumes questioning of whether the same ethical standards are applied in Africa compared to Europe or North America and suspicion that researchers and their sponsors take advantage of the lack of local legislation (Chima 2006) and weak social and health systems. These concerns have validity. For example, the Cameroon authorities stopped the trial of tenofovir, a drug being tested for HIV prevention, among female sex workers because the sponsors of the research did not provide treatment after the study (*Lancet* 2005).

Most publicly funded research proposals emanating from North America or Europe undergo stringent ethical reviews in the countries of origin and again, in the case of some African countries, in the countries where the research is to be conducted. However, one failing is that of omission. Such reviews presume capacity in the site locations or countries to monitor projects. Rarely is there consideration of the latent responsibility of the review boards to require researchers to take into account lack of local institutional capacity (for example, to provide support for local monitoring).[2]

A related consideration is the question of how researchers should address the threat of stigma and discrimination in studies on minority populations. There is need for sensitivity from the moment of planning a project through to dissemination of the results. On the one hand, such research can be important for providing reliable data about HIV infection among minority groups and influencing policy and programme agendas in terms of directing resources to people who otherwise might be ignored and who have difficulties accessing services (UNESCO 2002). On the other hand, the collection and publication of data on HIV among minority populations can contribute to discrimination against and within these populations (UNESCO 2002).

The use and abuse of histories of HIV and AIDS

A race-related issue that has pervaded public discourse on AIDS in sub-Saharan Africa is the origin of HIV. It should be noted that public discourse generally refers to the human immunodeficiency virus as a single entity. It ignores the scientific distinctions between two major types of the virus, HIV-1 and HIV-2, which have different epidemiologies (Greenberg et al. 2008).

The first case of HIV infection was formally defined in 1981 among a group of men who have sex with men (MSM) in the United States. However, some scientists have claimed that HIV was present in Africa for many decades preceding 1981. Greenberg and colleagues (2008) reported that the earliest known HIV-1 sero-positive specimens were identified through retrospective studies from Central Africa in 1959. HIV-2, which is believed to be less virulent than HIV-1, was first isolated in West Africa in the mid-1980s, but infection with this strain of HIV was said to have occurred in Guinea Bissau in the 1960s (Greenberg et al. 2008).

The portrayal of Africa as the site of origin of HIV inspired reactions among Africans ranging from outright denial in local press media to counter-arguments that since the first cases were found in the United States, Americans must have imported the virus into Africa through their 'abnormal' sexual practices, to claims that it was foreign propaganda to discourage investment in the continent (Lear 1998). In the 1980s, there were also reactions in Europe and North America – for example, calls for African students studying in foreign countries be tested for HIV, which led some editors of African newspapers, including the *Daily Times* in Nigeria, to call for a reciprocal policy to be adopted by the African Union, such that foreigners visiting Nigeria should also be tested for HIV before being allowed into the country. Adding fuel to the controversies, it must be remembered that the United States and Canada prohibited entry of HIV-positive persons to their countries (including international AIDS conferences held in those countries in the 1990s and early 2000s) until very recently.

The linking of racial identities with HIV has inevitably compounded racist perspectives in public discourse, inspiring what Bharat (2003) has characterised as 'double stigma' (racial stigma and stigma due to HIV/AIDS status). For example, in 1983 Haitian immigrants to the United States were prohibited from donating blood for fear of increasing the risk of HIV transmission within the American population via blood transfusions (Sabatier 1987). A recent Canadian study found that Africans and other immigrants who were HIV positive suffered racial discrimination (Gardezi et al. n.d.), which adversely resulted in poor health-seeking practices. Conversely, in 2008, it was reported that health officials in New Zealand were frustrated that African refugees who had been granted asylum and who were HIV positive were 'disappearing' into society and avoiding efforts to provide them with treatment. The officials' frustration stemmed, it was suggested, from their ignorance of the refugees' experiences of discrimination and, in particular, the refugees' knowledge of the stigma attached to HIV/AIDS in Africa, which would lead them to mistrust the health officials' actions.[3]

Race and gender

Race and gender are related themes that resonate in public discussions on HIV/AIDS and yet the latter has received more considered and sensitive accounting. Notably, the literature on gender has paid attention to the social constructs of sex and gender and how they influence trends in HIV epidemics. African scholars (for example, Adekunle and Ladipo 1992; Ajuwon and Shokunbi 1997; Kamau 2006), women's groups and international organisations (UNAIDS 2005) have recorded for many years that women in general, and African women in particular, are more vulnerable than men to being infected with HIV and to being negatively affected by HIV infections in their families and communities. In 2005, more than 77% of Africans living with HIV were women (UNAIDS 2005).

There are known biological and clinical explanations for the differential risk of infection between men and women in general. Women are three times more likely than men to become infected through sexual intercourse when they have sex with an infected person because the vaginal walls are delicate and prone to abrasion, which creates pathways for the transmission of HIV (Skejelmerud 1995). STIs, which are known to facilitate sexual transmission of HIV, are more difficult to diagnose in women than men. However, these factors are usually subsumed within analyses that draw attention to social and economic factors to explain the high rates of HIV infection amongst women.

The low social status of poor African women and their dependence on their male partners are well known as pervasive risk factors. For example, due to social conditioning and poverty, the majority of African women do not have control over the sexual behaviour of their male partners; the fidelity of a woman to her husband does not guarantee safety from infections because African men have the freedom to be adulterous while married women are expected to be absolutely faithful to their spouses and, as a consequence, a high proportion of married women acquire STIs from their spouses (Elemile 1992; Ajuwon and Shokunbi 1997; Van Niekerk 2002). Similarly, the links between poverty, social inequalities and involvement of women in risky occupations including sex work, itinerant hawking and apprenticeships in which they are subjected to sexual exploitation, are other known risk factors (Orubuloye, Caldwell and Caldwell 1993; Adekunle and Ladipo 1992; Ajuwon and Shokunbi 1997).

Notably, there has been research showing the linkage between sexual violence (including coercive sexual intercourse stemming from unequal power relations in relationships) and HIV infection among African women (Watts et al. 1998; Cáceres, Vanoss and Hudes 2000; Maman et al. 2001). For example, a study from Rwanda found that women who had experienced forced sex were significantly more likely than those with no history of forced sex to be infected with HIV (Van der Staten et al. 1998). Unfortunately, African women who had experienced violence perpetrated by spouses were likely to endure this behaviour because of the pervading belief that problems encountered in marriage are to be endured (Odujirin 1993; Adegbite 2005).

The inequities experienced by women begin earlier in their youth and are reflected in statistical estimates. For example, in South Africa, among the 15–24 year olds, young women account for 90% of new infections (UNAIDS/WHO 2008). The reasons are the same as those outlined above: in sum, a function of the relative powerlessness of women in society throughout Africa. Past and recent studies of girls involved in apprenticeship in informal trades in Africa capture the nature of these inequities (Sweat and Denison 1995; Dada, Olaseha and Ajuwon 1998; Ajuwon et al. 2002; Fawole et al. 2002; Fawole, Ajuwon and Osungbade 2004). One study from Nigeria found that many apprentice tailors reported unpaid labour, sexual harassment and reliance on exchanging sex for money to meet material needs (Ajuwon et al. 2002). Similar situations were reported among young female hawkers (Fawole et al. 2002).

The contrast between the discourse (public and scientific) on race and on gender in relation to HIV/AIDS is remarkable for the different directions taken in efforts to explain biophysical patterns in the transmission of HIV/AIDS. They run as if in parallel, the irony being that so little use has been made of the principles of gender-oriented studies to confront the misinformation that prevails with regard to race and HIV/AIDS.

Conclusion
Race and ethnicity are perennial themes in public and scientific explanations of the spread of HIV/AIDS in Africa. There are no known biological reasons to explain why racial or ethnic factors alone should alter the risk of STIs or HIV infection, which begs the question as to the purpose and value of attributing links between them. Africans may – indeed must – continue to confront the confusion caused by the ways in which race and ethnicity are linked to HIV/AIDS. However, the perpetuation of the racial and racist discourse within Africa reveals that Africans have yet to come to terms with the reality of HIV/AIDS on the continent. HIV/AIDS is still seen as a problem amongst this or that other population, thereby helping to perpetuate stigma and silence within families and communities. Gender-oriented studies to date show ways to break through what amounts to denial of this reality.

Notes

1. This category stems from convoluted political discourses in South Africa related to apartheid and attempts since 1994 to redress its inequities. The category 'African' is a politically expedient means to differentiate the category 'black', which can be read to include 'Indian' and 'Coloured'. It is a problematic distinction for serving primarily racially exclusive political agendas about who is or may be categorised as 'African'.
2. In 2007, a senior official in a South African provincial department of health complained about the inability of the department to monitor clinical trials because of the lack of vehicles within the department to visit sites and the burdensome bureaucratic procedures to obtain a vehicle (personal communication with T. Quinlan).
3. Personal communication with Judith King: Centre for Economic Governance and AIDS, Cape Town.

References

Adegbite, O. 2005. 'Intimate Partner Violence among Women of Child Bearing Age in Alimosho Local Government Area, Lagos, Nigeria'. Master of Public Health thesis. Ibadan: University of Ibadan.

Adekunle, A.O. and O. Ladipo. 1992. 'Reproductive Tract Infections in Nigeria: Challenges for a Fragile Health Infrastructure'. In K. Germain, P. Piot and R. Wasserhelt (eds). *Reproductive Tract Infections: Global Impact and Priorities for Women's Reproductive Health.* New York: Plenum Press: 297–315.

Ajuwon, A., W. McFarland, E. Hudes, S. Adedapo, T. Okikiolu and P. Lurie. 2002. 'HIV Risk-Related Behavior, Sexual Coercion, and Implications for Prevention Strategies among Female Apprentice Tailors in Ibadan, Nigeria'. *AIDS and Behavior* 6(3): 229–35.

Ajuwon, A. and W. Shokunbi. 1997. 'Women and the Risk of HIV Infection in Nigeria: Implications for Control Programs'. *International Quarterly of Community Health Education* 17: 102–20.

Auvert, B., D. Taljaard, E. Lagarde, J. Sobngwi-Tambekou, R. Sitta and A. Puren. 2005. 'Randomised, Controlled Intervention Trial of Male Circumcision for Reduction of HIV Infection Risk: The ANRS 1265 Trial'. *PLoS Medicine* 2(11): 2 298.

Bailey, R.C., S. Moses, C.B. Parker, K. Agot, I. Maclean, J.N. Krieger, C.F.M. Williams, R.T. Campbell and J.O. Ndinya-Achola. 2007. 'Male Circumcision for HIV Prevention in Young Men in Kisuma, Kenya: A Randomised Controlled Trial'. *Lancet* 369(9562): 643–56.

Bharat, S. 2003. *Racism, Racial Discrimination and Related Intolerance Relating to HIV/AIDS.* Paris: UNESCO.

Bhopal, R. 1997. 'Is Research into Ethnicity and Health Racist, Unsound, or Important Science?' *British Medical Journal* 3(14): 1751-6.

Cáceres, C., M. Vanoss and E. Hudes. 2000. 'Sexual Coercion among Youth and Young Adults in Lima, Peru'. *Journal of Adolescent Health* 27(5): 361-7.

CDC (Center for Disease Control and Prevention). 2008. 'HIV/AIDS among African Americans'. Fact sheet. Available at www.cdc.gov/hiv/topics/aa/.

Chima, S. 2006. 'Regulation of Biomedical Research in Africa'. *British Medical Journal* 332: 848-51.

Dada, J., I. Olaseha and A. Ajuwon. 1998. 'Sexual Behaviour and Knowledge of AIDS among Female Trade Apprentices in a Yoruba Town in South-Western Nigeria'. *International Quarterly of Community Health Education* 17(3): 255-70.

Dilraj, A., S. Abdool Karim and S. Pillay. 2007. 'Challenging Racial Stereotyping of AIDS in South Africa with Prevalence of HIV in Pregnant Women'. *South African Medical Journal* 7(1): 43-4.

Dougan, S., L. Payne, A. Brown, K. Fenton, L. Logan, B. Evans and O. Gill. 2004. 'Black Caribbean Adults with HIV in England, Wales, and Northern Ireland: An Emerging Epidemic?' *Sexually Transmitted Infections* 80: 18-23.

Dunn, C. and M. Chadwick. 1999. 'Protecting Study Volunteers in Research'. Available at www.centerwatch.com.

Elemile, T. 1992. 'The Epidemiology of Sexually Transmitted Diseases in a Rural Area, Ilora, Oyo State, Nigeria'. Post-graduate fellowship dissertation of the National College of Public Health.

Fawole O., A. Ajuwon and K. Osungbade. 2004. 'Violence and HIV/AIDS Prevention among Female Out-of-School Youths in South-Western Nigeria: Lessons Learnt from Interventions Targeted at Hawkers and Apprentices'. *African Journal of Medicine and Medical Sciences* 33: 347-53.

Fawole, O., A. Ajuwon, K. Osungbade and O. Faweya. 2002. 'Prevalence of Violence against Young Female Hawkers in Three Cities in Southwestern Nigeria'. *Health Education* 102(5): 230-8.

Fenton, K., A. Johnson and A. Nicoll. 1997. 'Race, Ethnicity, and Sexual Health'. *British Medical Journal* 314: 1703.

FMOH (Federal Ministry of Health), Nigeria. 2006. *National Sero-Prevalence Sentinel Survey*. Abuja: Federal Ministry of Health.

Gardezi, F., L. Calzavara, E. Lawson, W. Husbands, E. Tharao, D. Willms, C. George, T. Meyers, R. Rennis, D. Taylor, S. Adebajo, F. McGee and E.J. Wambayi. n.d. 'Racism and HIV/AIDS: Impacts of Racialized Discourse on the Daily Lives of Africans and Carribean Communities in Toronto, Canada'. Unpublished report.

Gray, R.H., G. Kigozi, D. Serwada, F. Makumbi, S. Watya, F. Nalugoda, N. Kiwanuka, L.W. Moulton, M.A. Chaudhary, M.Z. Chen, N.K. Sewankambo, F. Wabwire-Manengen, M.C. Bacon, C.F.M. Williams, P. Opendi, S.T. Reynolds, O. Laeyendecker, T.C. Quinn and M. Wawer. 2007. 'Male Circumcision for HIV Prevention in Young Men in Rakai, Uganda: A Randomized Trial'. *Lancet* 369: 657-66.

Greenberg, A., P. Drotman, J. Curran and R. Janssen. 2008. 'The Epidemiology of Human Immunodeficiency Virus Infection and Acquired Immunodeficiency Syndrome'. In R.B. Wallace and N. Kohatsu (eds). *Public Health and Preventive Medicine*. New York: McGraw Hill: 189–200.

Guenter, D., J. Esparza and R. Macklin. 2000. 'Ethical Considerations in HIV Vaccine Trials: Summary of a Consultative Process Conducted by the Joint United Nations Programme on HIV/AIDS (UNAIDS)'. *Journal of Medical Ethics* 26(1): 37–47.

Kamau, N. 2006. 'Invisibility, Silence and Absence: A Study of the Account Taken by Two Kenyan Universities of the Effects of HIV and AIDS on Senior Women Staff'. *Women's Studies International Forum* 29: 612–19.

Lacey, C., D. Merrick, D. Bensley and I. Fairley. 1997. 'Analysis of the Socio-demography of Gonorrhoea in Leeds'. *British Medical Journal* 314: 1715–18.

Lancet. 2005. 'The Trials of Tenofovir Trials'. *Lancet* 365: 1111.

Landis, J. 1974. *Sociology: Concepts and Characteristics*. Wadsworth: Belmont.

Lear, D. 1998. 'AIDS in the African Press'. In D. Buchanan and G. Cernada (eds). *Progress in Preventing AIDS? Dogma, Dissent and Innovation*. Amityville: Baywood Press: 215–25.

Lurie, P. and S. Wolfe. 1997. 'Unethical Trials of Interventions to Reduce Perinatal Transmission of the Human Immunodeficiency Virus in Developing Countries'. *New England Journal of Medicine* 337: 853–6.

Maman, S., J. Mbwanbo, M. Hogan, G. Kilonzo, M. Sweat and E. Weiss. 2001. *HIV and Partner Violence: Implications for HIV Voluntary Counseling and Testing Programmes in Dar es Salaam*. New York: Population Council.

Marshall, W. 2005. 'Aids, Race and the Limits of Science'. *Social Science and Medicine* 60: 2 515–25.

Metam. 2008. 'Summary of Provincial HIV and AIDS Statistics for South Africa'. October. Available at www.metam.co.za.

NIBUCAA (Nigerian Business Coalition Against AIDS). 2007. 'Document on Call for Proposal'. Lagos: NIBUCAA.

Odujirin, O. 1993. 'Domestic Violence among Married Women in Lagos'. *International Journal of Gynaecology and Obstetrics* 34: 361–66.

O'Neil, D. 2008. *Ethnicity and Race: An Introduction to the Nature and Social Group Differentiation and Inequality*. San Marcos: Palomar College.

Orubuloye, I., P. Caldwell and J. Caldwell. 1993. 'The Role of High-Risk Occupations in the Spread of AIDS: Truck Drivers and Itinerant Market Women in Nigeria'. *International Family Planning Perspectives* 19: 43–8.

Quinn, T., M. Wawer, N. Sewankambo, D. Serwadda, C. Li, F. Wabwire-Mangen, M.O. Meehan, T. Lutalo and R. Gray. 2000. 'Viral Load and Heterosexual Transmission of Human Immunodeficiency Virus Type 1'. *New England Journal of Medicine* 342(13): 921–9.

Sabatier, R. 1987. 'Social, Cultural and Demographic Aspects of AIDS'. *Western Journal of Medicine* 147(6): 713–15.

Skejelmerud, A. 1995. 'Women in the AIDS Crisis'. *Contact Magazine* 144: 3-5.

Springer, C. 1998. 'Sociology of AIDS within the Black Communities: Theoretical Considerations'. In D. Buchanan and G. Cernada (eds). *Progress in Preventing AIDS? Dogma, Dissent and Innovation.* Amityville: Baywood Press: 203-14.

St Louis, M., T. Farley and S. Aral. 1996. 'Untangling the Persistence of Syphilis in the South'. *Sexually Transmitted Diseases* 23: 1-4.

Sweat, M. and J. Denison. 1995. 'Reducing HIV Incidence in Developing Countries with Structural and Environmental Interventions'. *AIDS* 9: S251-S257.

UNAIDS (Joint United Nations Programme on HIV/AIDS). 2005. 'AIDS Epidemic Update'. Geneva: UNAIDS.

———. 2009. 'Sub-Saharan Africa, Fact Sheet No. 9'. Geneva: UNAIDS.

UNAIDS/WHO (World Health Organization). 2008. 'Sub-Saharan Africa AIDS Epidemic Update, Regional Summary'. Geneva: UNAIDS and WHO.

UNESCO (United Nations Educational, Cultural and Scientific Organization). 2002. 'The Millennium Development Goals and Indigenous People: Redefining the Goals'. Paris: UNESCO.

Van der Staten, A., R. King, O. Grinstead, E. Vittinghoff, A. Serufillira and S. Allen. 1998. 'Sexual Coercion, Physical Violence and HIV Infection among Women in Steady Relationships in Kigali, Rwanda'. *AIDS and Behavior* 2(1): 61-72.

Van Niekerk, A. 2002. 'Moral and Social Complexities of AIDS in Africa'. *Journal of Medicine and Philosophy* 27(2): 143-62.

Wanyenze, R., C. Nawavvu, A. Namale, A. Mayanja, R. Bunnell, B. Abang, G. Amanyire, N. Sewankambo and M. Kamya. 2008. 'Acceptability of Routine HIV Counselling and Testing, and HIV Seroprevalence in Ugandan Hospitals'. *Bulletin of the World Health Organization* 86(4): 302-9.

Watts C., E. Keogh, M. Ndlovu and R. Kwaramba. 1998. 'Withholding Sex and Forced Sex: Dimensions of Violence against Zimbabwean Women'. *Reproductive Health Matters* 6(12): 57-65.

10

The Politics of AIDS in South Africa

Foundations of a Hyperendemic Epidemic

Warren Parker

The politics of AIDS in South Africa has to do with understanding how the disease has unfolded epidemiologically in relation to inequalities of political power grounded in socio-economic disparities. According to statistics from the Actuarial Society of South Africa and the Joint United Nations Programme on HIV/AIDS (UNAIDS), by 2007 South Africa's HIV epidemic was one-sixth of the global total of infections (5.5 million of a total of 33.2 million), in spite of a stable post-liberation government and a relatively advanced economy. It seems inexplicable that South Africa should have so disproportionate a share of the global burden of HIV. Many of the building blocks for an adequate response to the disease were put in place in the post-apartheid era: a large governmental and non-governmental HIV/AIDS service sector, endorsement of the principle of multisectoral response and multibillion-dollar donor commitments. Clearly multiple intersecting factors have been at play and, in seeking understanding, two questions emerge: What particular factors contributed to South Africa's disproportionate share of the global HIV burden, and is it possible to reverse this trend?

At a macro-level, factors include political meddling and intransigence, global AIDS policies and guidelines that do not take into account country-specific contexts, funding regimes that are overly centralised and anti-developmental and linkages between globalisation, urbanisation, mobility and poverty. At a micro-level, factors include multiple concurrent sexual partnerships, which create densely clustered sexual networks that are fostered by inequality and marginalisation. Additionally, the under-resourcing of grassroots organisations hinders the country's support for prevention and care efforts. This chapter argues for leadership and mobilisation that recognises that people's vulnerability to infection is a product of socio-economic factors and eschews political and economic elitism in favour of grassroots-focused policies and practices.

Sexual networks and HIV risk

The rapid growth of HIV infection in South Africa has been concommitant with sexual networks that are closely interwoven and link HIV-positive and -negative individuals. These networks underlie family structures and communal values and norms. They exist in a context of a highly mobile population in conjunction with a breakdown of social regulation of sexual interactions. The emergence of these sexual networks is connected to historically rooted economic factors – notably, apartheid-era male labour migration driven by the mining industry and expanding urban industrialisation. Such migration fostered a pattern of geographically diversified sexual networks that provided fertile ground for the spread of HIV when the disease appeared in South Africa in the 1980s. The early trajectory of HIV was thus largely amongst migrant miners, with further infections occurring in the communities to which the migrants perennially returned.

The transition to the new democratic order in the 1990s held a promise that HIV infections driven by inequality and marginalisation would be curtailed. However, the post-apartheid era has witnessed a magnification of the problem as a result of the liberalisation of rights to freedom of movement and residence. Rural-urban mobility and mobility in general has accelerated as a result of people being free to seek formal employment wherever they wish and it has also resulted in the burgeoning of a class of unemployed who earn small incomes in the informal sector. Women's general greater risk of infection, due to their biological and socio-cultural vulnerabilities, has been exacerbated by greater mobility. One known outcome of these conditions is that income-generation strategies can include transactional sex for material gain.

The movement of people to urban centres, in combination with limited availability of housing and pervasive poverty and unemployment, led to a rapid growth of informal settlements on the periphery of most towns and cities. These vast shacklands are characterised by fluctuating populations, social fragmentation, relatively poor access to water, electricity and sanitation and poorly developed civic structures.[1] Fluid and overlapping sexual relationships flourish in these conditions. For instance, residents of informal settlements are more likely to report having two or more sexual partners in the past year than people living in other forms of settlement. Being exposed to multiple sexual partners is associated with increased risk of HIV infection (Shisana et al. 2005). Therefore, it is no surprise that surveys of HIV prevalence in South Africa have found considerably higher levels of HIV infection in informal settlements than in rural or formal urban areas (Shisana et al. 2005).

Urbanisation and the growth of informal settlements provide one example of how historically grounded economic practices shift over time in ways that increase the risk of HIV infection. However, the epidemic is not exclusive to marginalised communities; HIV weaves through the nation, leading to diverse patterns of infection and on the basis of diverse vulnerabilities amongst different sub-populations. That said, it is the poor and marginalised who are most vulnerable and the scale of South Africa's epidemic has much to do with a failure to address pathways of risk and the structural economics of vulnerability.

A fractured response

Initial responses to AIDS in South Africa occurred in the late phase of the apartheid era and were roundly criticised by the progressive African National Congress (ANC)-aligned health movement. In particular, criticism was levelled at racial stereotyping in the different AIDS 'messages' directed at 'white' and 'non-white' audiences (Parker et al.

2007). In contrast, the progressive health movement, a collective of non-governmental organisations (NGOs), largely resourced through foreign funding and supported through a combination of structures falling within the ambit of the mass democratic movement, convened the National AIDS Committee of South Africa (NACOSA). NACOSA was instrumental in developing South Africa's first national AIDS plan in the early 1990s, a plan that was intended to form the basis for a post-apartheid era response to the epidemic (Butler 2005: 593).

However, donor policies changed following the transition to an ANC-led government. Donor resources were rapidly withdrawn from the leading NGOs of the time, including health service-oriented organisations. Funds were directed instead towards bilateral and other arrangements with the new government. Consequently, many formerly robust organisations shrank or disappeared (Schneider and Stein 2001).

In the post-apartheid era, optimism about government leadership on AIDS rapidly diminished. Nelson Mandela deferred leadership on the issue to the then health minister, Nkosazana Dlamini-Zuma, and the deputy president, Thabo Mbeki. The NACOSA plan had provided a foundation for a new response to the epidemic, but an inept investment by the Department of Health in an overly expensive and poorly conceptualised AIDS play, *Sarafina! 2*, signalled the start of a series of politically charged forays into the margins of AIDS policy and practice. The collective wisdom of the NACOSA plan was set aside in favour of pursuits of fancy, such as an indigenous AIDS 'cure' named Virodene (Schneider and Stein 2001) and the contrarian musings of Mbeki who suggested that HIV did not cause AIDS (in the process romancing and legitimating a small band of American scientists who laboured under the banner of AIDS denialism) (Schneider and Fassin 2002). The next health minister, Manto Tshabalala-Msimang, sowed more seeds of doubt with the tacit support of the Mbeki government. Notably, she disparaged drug therapies for the prevention of mother-to-child HIV transmission and antiretroviral (ARV) treatment for people with advanced HIV infection.

There is little doubt that this intransigence led to the unnecessary infection of tens of thousands of babies, many of whom died in early infancy, and many more parents and relatives struggling with the trauma of loss. Indeed, a modelling analysis of AIDS deaths estimated that more than 330 000 lives were lost as a consequence of government policy between 2000 and 2005 (Chigwedere et al. 2008; Nattrass 2004). Similarly, for older children and adults living with HIV, life-extending drugs were denied for several years – government obduracy ending only as a result of the active resistance of the Treatment Action Campaign and allied groups and court judgements (Willan 2004).

Although Mbeki and Tshabalala-Msimang were sceptical about ARVs, the national government initiated other orthodox interventions with considerable success. For example, it put in place a robust public-sector condom distribution programme (more than 300 million condoms per annum) and voluntary counselling and testing (VCT) services at many clinics and hospitals. Initial reports suggested that levels of condom use (reported use at last sexual encounter) and HIV testing had increased (Shisana et al. 2005). There was a gradual expansion in non-governmental interventions, largely amongst relatively small organisations working at community level with the immediate exigencies of the epidemic, as well as growth in workplace programmes in the private sector. Further afield, there were shifts in global strategy and policy led by various United Nations bodies. These included centralisation of funding within The Global Fund to Fight AIDS, Tuberculosis and Malaria (GFATM) and a focus on Africa in which the United States played a leading role via the President's Emergency Plan for AIDS Relief (PEPFAR).

Much of the rhetoric of the international agencies emphasised centralised programming at national government level, supported by massive amounts of money. GFATM focused on streaming resources through government-led Country Co-ordinating Mechanisms (CCMs) and PEPFAR emphasised service delivery through governmental and non-governmental structures and organisations. South Africa received massive commitments in the first round of GFATM proposals in 2002, including $68 million over five years for the loveLife programme and $62 million for provincial-level HIV/AIDS care and support in KwaZulu-Natal.

By 2005, the South African government's investment in HIV/AIDS had increased significantly and most of the internationally approved policy and programmatic building blocks were in place. These included continued support to free condom distribution and VCT services, alongside the provision of ARV treatment and legislation that endorsed a human rights approach to people living with HIV/AIDS. Local non-governmental interventions had secured massive funding support from provincial governments, the corporate sector, local and international foundations and donor countries.

By the end of 2008, billions had cumulatively been expended on the epidemic with efforts spanning government, the formal 'AIDS industry' and other less formalised responses. By this time and by the standards of global discourse, most of the bases were covered. South Africa was by and large 'doing the right thing'. Yet the country's epidemic showed little sign of abating.

The dislocation of local response

There is much to be said about the failure of the global discourse that has underpinned and framed South Africa's HIV/AIDS strategies and policies. Notably, it does not necessarily follow that the direction of thinking within international bureaucracies adequately considers the needs and contexts of affected communities. Many of the early lessons in HIV prevention were quickly abandoned in favour of a growth in bureaucratic structures aligned around massive financial resources that did little to transform the social and economic conditions in the poor communities who have borne the brunt of the epidemic.

For instance, non-governmental services were typically bracketed by short-term funding for projects on predetermined areas of focus. The PEPFAR programme, for example, provided $855 million to South Africa between 2004 and 2007 to achieve targets defined in terms of numbers of people reached by services and activities conducted. This was the basis on which it could claim effectiveness in key areas such as the provision of ARVs, caregiving, support to orphans, prevention of mother-to-child transmission and VCT.[2] However, these achievements do not consider effectiveness in terms of actual, regular use of condoms, for example, or proportion of individuals of the total who get tested and who change their behaviour or, as necessary, subscribe to ARVs, adhere to treatment regimes and, as importantly, success rates in terms of numbers of people still alive after one and more years of receiving treatment.

In counterpoint, one of the first examples of a successful reversal of a severe epidemic can be found in the gay community in the United States during the 1980s. The response, in context of the mysterious spread of HIV amongst gay men, saw mobilisation of a range of grassroots strategies to combat the disease. 'Gay bath houses', where anonymous sex and promiscuity were common, were shut down. Gay men mobilised in street demonstrations to raise awareness and to encourage government attention. There was close collaboration between medical and social researchers and the affected community. Posters, information leaflets and condoms were distributed widely. 'Support groups' and 'buddy' programmes were set up to help those living with HIV as well as the ill and bereaved. Downward trends in infection were soon evident (Shilts 2000; Crimp and Rolston 1990). Similarly, Uganda succeeded in curtailing an HIV/AIDS epidemic in the late 1980s and early 1990s. The response included decisive political and civic leadership at national and grassroots levels, coupled with community responses that focused on changing patterns of sexual relationships (with a particular emphasis on reducing multiple sexual partnerships) in conjunction with support to affected individuals and families (Low-Beer and Stoneburner 2004; Green et al. 2006).

In neither the United States nor Uganda, were these successes based on massive resources and bureaucracies. There was no big money, no top-down structures, no multilayered policy or strategy documents and no sea of consultants and experts advising on what was to be done. Yet in both instances, HIV-infection patterns were markedly reversed (Green et al. 2006; Shilts 2000). In both cases, there were distinct shifts in the political sphere; in the United States, prioritisation of the epidemic within government programming; in Uganda, embracing of the perceived need to mobilise society as a whole. A common significant feature was the prominent location of response at grassroots level, amongst and within affected communities themselves.

Yet globally, there has been little indication of support to use that lesson. Instead, as is the case in South Africa, the most severely affected communities remain marginalised in favour of an international and national bureaucracy that sets the agenda, defines activities, specifies funding mechanisms and determines 'outputs'. There is virtually no attention given to empowerment of local actors. Community mobilisation on the basis of a plethora of small community-based organisations (CBOs) occurs widely, but it is drastically under-resourced. Consider, for example, the following quotes drawn from interviews with community-based organisations (Makhubele and Parker 2008):

> When we were established we operated without funding. I was responsible for everything in the organisation, even using my own money to get necessities like food and clothing for the children (director, children's project, Western Cape).

> I think funders have a particular ideology on how programmes should be implemented. They want the money to be used to implement activities, but these activities need to be run by skilled staff who are paid sufficiently to enable them to manage these activities. So that is the mind-shift that is required. You can't just fund the activities without funding and supporting the people who manage them (AIDS networking organisation, Cape Town).

> Because of the skills they have acquired, some have been taken as lay counsellors by government because of their training . . . We groom them, but they are taken by others because they promise higher salaries . . . That is our challenge (director, home-based care organisation, Limpopo).

> You may find a patient living in an inhospitable household where there is no food. The caregiver will sacrifice some of their stipend to buy food for the patient . . . Sometimes there are patients who are unable to walk to clinics, and caregivers will use their own money for transport (home-based care organisation, Limpopo).

These reflections illustrate the alienation and marginalisation of community-based responses to HIV. Organic responses are funded by committed individuals who gradually secure external funding. Interest and commitment abound at community level, often driven by the visible exigencies and lived experience of the epidemic, but there is usually no external support structure to help harness local endeavours. In our research, respondents voiced their lack of capacity to write funding proposals and their lack of knowledge on how to identify potential funders, let alone to frame proposals in accordance with the many different regulations and orientations of different funding agencies. They struggle to secure resources and support for organisational and personnel development. There is underfunding of salaries to the extent that trained staff are likely to be 'cherry-picked' by government and other organisations once they have built up a repertoire of skills (Makhubele and Parker 2008). There is a skewed reliance on cadres of volunteers to bridge the gaps in services supported by donors. For example, donors often provide funding for ARVs, but not for food or transport for patients on the drugs. Furthermore, funding regimes for smaller organisations rely on the absurd notion that already impoverished communities can provide volunteers who can earn stipends that are well below the breadline.

The final quote above particularly underscores the myopic misallocation of resources through the global AIDS machinery. What can one conclude from a situation where local and global AIDS elites move between conferences, workshops and action plans whilst community-based volunteers commit their meagre stipends to patients under their care for food and transport?

Commodification of sex and the epidemiology of HIV

The distribution of HIV globally and the varying growth rates of epidemics at country level have much to do with the nature of underlying political and economic factors and how they intersect. It has become apparent, for example, that significant epidemics have occurred mainly in sub-Saharan Africa and that so-called hyperendemic or severe epidemics are occurring only in southern Africa. The conventional wisdom on HIV prevention, commonly exemplified under the banner of ABC (Abstain, Be Faithful, Condomise), has been applied in southern Africa, but it clearly has not worked. Lack of empirical understanding of the factors underpinning the epidemic and limited engagement with key elements that increase risk of and vulnerability to infection are key reasons for this failure.

One of the first layers of risk relates to economic disparity within poor communities, where the unemployed and poor reside alongside marginally better-off, employed residents. It is here that a prominent pattern of exchange of sex for economic and other benefits has emerged. And it is this pattern that contributes significantly to densely clustered sexual networks that accentuate the risk of HIV infection (Halperin and Epstein 2007). The following quotes are drawn from a series of interviews and discussions with young adults living in an informal settlement near Johannesburg (Hajiyiannis and Parker 2008). They illustrate the inequalities and power differentials that provide a pathway for what is formally defined as 'transactional sex':

> [Sex] is a passport to clothing and finance. Older men have all the care in this world. It is why a woman needs to have sugar daddies in order to survive. And it makes me feel like a natural woman. That is why I love sugar daddies cause they always say yes to whatever young girls need (female discussant, Orange Farm).

> I am 23 years old, I'm married with a 27-year-old woman and we have a 5-month-old boy. I lost my job two years back. I was forced to find someone to help me in supporting my family. She's old and she helps me very much and she enjoys my service such as my sex experience. My wife doesn't know what is happening. I always tell her that I am finding piece jobs (male discussant, Orange Farm).

Hunter (2002) distinguishes between sex for subsistence and sex for consumption; both are common amongst those who are unemployed.

Personal 'needs' are not always the only needs being addressed; for some, there is an altruistic function where exchange benefits other family members. Of epidemiological importance is that these sexual relationships, irrespective of the motivation, often involve multiple and overlapping sexual partners. When sexual relationships overlap in this way, the result is a relatively open sexual network with numerous channels for the transmission of HIV. In addition, there is one important factor that affects the pace of transmission. When a person is newly infected, the virus replicates rapidly, leading to a high viral load in bodily fluids, which increases the probability of transmission in a sexual encounter. The probability of infection is at least ten times more likely than when a person is in the middle phase or latent phase of infection – meaning that the viral load diminishes over time and, with treatment, can become negligible (Morris and Kretzschmar 2000; Latora et al. 2006).[3]

Poverty is, of course, a link in the transmission of HIV. Indeed, even President Mbeki was aware of this link when he suggested that poverty 'caused AIDS' whilst propounding doubts about viral transmission of HIV. Aside from his simplistic assessment, his observation did not lead to any substantive review or change in his government's AIDS policy and programmes. Instead, his government continued to commit billions of dollars to an arms deal and to entrench the economic policy of Growth, Employment and Redistribution (GEAR) to supplant the Reconstruction and Development Programme (RDP), which, in the mid-1990s, had demonstrated the national government's commitment to poverty alleviation.

A glaring gap in the formal AIDS response

National HIV/AIDS policies are largely a product of a 'boilerplate' model of intervention that is assumed to be applicable to all HIV epidemics. For example, national AIDS plans are regarded as necessary to secure donor funding. National reporting on epidemics consists largely of checklists for interventions that are considered tried and tested and 'the right thing to do'. However, there is little emphasis on deep analysis of the epidemiology of HIV/AIDS within countries and, consequently, little sequencing and prioritisation of interventions. The absence of adequate strategic analysis embedded in national plans diminishes the possibility of meeting ambitious goals and targets. South Africa's AIDS policies and plans generally align well with international guidelines. However, the fact remains that the country has failed to significantly reduce new HIV infections in the first two decades of the epidemic. There were and still are major gaps in the national response, which I outline below.

With regard to the key risk factor – exposure to HIV infection via sexual networks – there has been a distinct failure to communicate the threat in ways that are relevant to those who are at risk. Communication campaigns have created high levels awareness of the importance of condom use, but not about the risks of having multiple and overlapping sexual partners. A national study in 2006 amongst unmarried 20–30-year-olds found that 94% of the informants mentioned using condoms, but only 22% mentioned sticking to one partner and when asked what ways they knew of to prevent HIV, only 5% mentioned reducing or limiting their number of partners (Parker et al. 2007). Furthermore, there has been little consideration of how to formulate key prevention measures and principles for behaviour change in the messages conveyed by research and communication campaigns. Faithfulness, for example, has been a cornerstone of how monogamy might be communicated but it has failed as a prevention concept within South African communities at risk. The quotes below from a national study on sexual relationships illustrate that the concept of faithfulness does not necessarily mean monogamy; instead, it has alternate meanings in some high-risk populations in the country:

> Being faithful is protecting the one you love from hurt. You make sure that he only knows the best about you and you give him the best love. The others are just there when he is not around, to keep you company (focus group discussion, females 20–30, Gauteng).

> As for me I have my girlfriend, the one that I spend most of my time with. I am faithful to her because even when I have other

girlfriends I do not walk around with them for her to see me. I hide the other girlfriends (focus group discussion, males 20–30, Gauteng) (Parker et al. 2007).

These were not atypical comments. Focus group participants in multiple sites described a predominant pattern of having 'main' and 'other' partners: the 'main' partner being the person one loved; 'other' partners being the outcome of sexual desire or material benefit. Many participants mentioned condom use as an important method for HIV prevention, but also indicated that condom use decreased within quite short periods of time with 'main' sexual partners and was inconsistent with 'other' sexual partners (Parker et al. 2007). Likewise, cohabiting and marriage are not commonly subscribed foundations to reduce the likelihood of having concurrent sexual partners. Very few South Africans in their twenties and thirties are married or cohabiting and even amongst older adults (31–39), only half were estimated to be married or cohabiting in 2006 (Parker et al. 2007). These findings stand in contrast to the evident, initial success of campaigns in the past to change behaviour. By 2005, for example, 73% of males and 56% of females aged 15–24 who were sexually active reported using condoms at last sex; a marked change from a decade before where condom use was rare. Similarly, by 2005, 44% of people aged 25–49 had tested for HIV and, amongst this group, more than a third (37%) had been tested in the past year (Shisana et al. 2005). Unfortunately, neither condom use nor VCT has had any substantive effect on the phenomenon of concurrent sexual partnering. In particular, VCT has been propounded as a useful prevention intervention, but it has been found to have little impact on prevention amongst individuals who test HIV negative (Corbett et al. 2007).

In summary, condom use and VCT promotion have gained footing in populations at risk, but there has been little attention paid to a central epidemiological factor: multiple and overlapping sexual partnerships. This lack of focus has meant that concurrent sexual partnering has not been a 'top-of-mind' risk factor amongst South Africans.

The seductive nature of global values

Material consumption is a central feature of South African society and is often manifest in sexual relationships, more so where symbolic values of wealth are attached to visible ownership of commodities. Leclerc-Madlala (2004), like Hunter (2002), has observed the commodification of sex, whereby sexual partnerships of varying durations allow for the accumulation of goods and services. She has noted that subsistence 'needs' include food, rent, clothing, school fees and transport and merge with 'wants' such as cell phones, fashion items, tertiary education fees and luxury transport. Sex was openly acknowledged by young women in her study as a simple means to satisfy needs and wants.

Previously, these attitudes and practices amongst the youth were seen counterintuitively as an opportunity for an HIV-prevention intervention. The principle was that reification and consumption of branded goods could be a mechanism for building trust and promoting HIV prevention amongst the youth. The most notable experiment has been an investment of $20 million per annum in an HIV youth-focused project, loveLife, since the late 1990s. The programme was developed by the American Henry J. Kaiser Family Foundation and funded in partnership with the Bill and Melinda Gates Foundation, GFATM and the South African government. The programme propounded the merits of fostering individual optimism through consumption, which in turn was expected to promote HIV-risk reduction. As Kaiser Foundation president Drew Altman noted at a launch of a loveLife youth Y-Centre in the sprawling Orange Farm informal settlement in 2003:

> loveLife is not only big, but I think anybody who knows the programme would say that it is cutting edge, and it is bold and it is different. It is not just a safe sex campaign, though there are elements of that. It is not even just an HIV prevention campaign, but it is a national movement led by young people themselves about positive lifestyles and better futures (Naidoo 2003: 1).

However, this project failed to take into account the extent of poverty in the communities the programme was supposedly serving. In particular, it ignored the absence of resources amongst young residents to support a lifestyle of conspicuous material consumption that was seen as necessary to craft a pathway to HIV prevention. Instead, impoverished youth were well aware of the attempts to create a different class of youth in their midst; the Y-Centre simply accentuated differences between the small group of youth who were able to embrace the loveLife lifestyle and the poorer majority who could not:

> You know, they [loveLife members] are always in groups. Whenever they go to Y-Centre and whenever they come back. So, you know, one will think that okay . . . it's a specific group, so they've called them or they've sent in something, whilst you don't need a CV to go to a community centre. So, looking at them in a group, they are all dressed in expensive clothes and everything. So, as Orange Farm it's a very much poor area, so most people don't work. Young people feel that there's a tension between them because they can't afford to buy those expensive clothes they have there at Y-Centre.
>
> I think at Y-Centre most young people are affected by peer pressure . . . Peer pressure happens within the centre because if you don't have expensive clothes . . . you start pressurising your parents for more money, clothes, etc. (Naidoo 2003: 13).

The influence of globalisation and consumption on HIV risk is also multifarious. Consider cell phones, for example. They are sought-after commodities that have both practical application and aggrandise perceptions of economic status. However, cell phones and massive marketing of them has provided opportunities for accessing sexual partners in ways that were not possible fifteen years ago. As one young man stated: 'Once she gives you her numbers . . . it is already a contract [for sex]' (Parker et al. 2007: 29). In addition, the mass media (for example, films, drama series and soap operas), often with formulaic plot themes emanating from the North, have had a negative influence on South African youth, but the relationship in the context of HIV/ AIDS has not been addressed significantly. Again, comments in a focus group discussion, illustrate the point:

> Male 1: You look at *Days of Our Lives* and *Generations* . . . When you look at what is shown in *Days* for example . . . This one gets married to this one, the stepmother is married to the father but has an affair with her stepson. The stepson has an affair with the stepsister . . .

> Male 2: Those are the things that are causing a lot of confusion in our communities . . . They are written in such a way that they grip your attention . . .[4]

While not necessarily directly causal, the effect of such programming is to legitimate particular practices, in the above instance, promiscuity. This is significant in a context where HIV projects and programmes targeting the youth do not confront the influence and do not prioritise the risks of concurrent sexual partnering. In South Africa, poverty and inequality intersects with broadcasting of symbols purporting to allow transcendence of poverty (for example, cell phone ownership, fashionable dress, access to transport) and of messages that venerate the sexual lifestyles of the other (as exemplified in soap operas). The outcome is confusion and doubt at best amongst young people, as indicated in the quotes above and, at worst, legitimation of value systems that are contrary to those propounded in HIV-prevention campaigns.

Drawing together the strands
South Africa's disproportionate contribution to the global total of people living with HIV is the result in part of a distinct lack of political leadership and ineffective mobilisation of the population. In this chapter I have focused on the escalation of HIV infection in South Africa. I have argued that a range of intersecting political and economic factors underpins a socio-cultural environment that has encouraged the reproduction – rather than reduction – of the HIV epidemic.

AIDS is a complex and insidious disease that moves slowly through communities and societies. South Africa is an example of how it often fails to prompt concerted and co-ordinated action. The disease has been diminished in communities and societies where there has been such action, at least in the short to medium term. The lesson learned is that political and social mobilisation within affected communities is essential. The responses of the gay community in the United States and Uganda's early successes are examples.

There was potential for mobilisation in South Africa in that communities could have built on their experiences of struggle and resistance during the apartheid era to address AIDS. However, this did not happen. The potential faded in the face of the economic marginalisation that is a characteristic of heightened risk and vulnerability to HIV infection. People have become more mobile. Communities have become fragmented. Mechanisms of community leadership and accountability have shifted.

The seeds for effective mobilisation clearly exist within communities as is testified by the existence of many CBOs that confront different aspects of the epidemic, such as home-based patient care, orphan care and counselling. But it is this response that has been marginalised by funding and programming regimes dictated by national and international bureaucracies; indeed, there is little evidence of political and strategic recognition of the importance of grassroots formations. Reinvigorating community response requires political action. At national level this requires the legitimation of community mobilisation and leadership in response to the epidemic, whilst at community level there is a need for leadership that harnesses community resources and government and NGO services and capacities.

There is a major challenge at the international level. The politics of AIDS is framed by bureaucracy and paternalism. Funding is centralised. Models for intervention are standardised. Governments and large organisations are given priority. Accountability is finessed by numerical facts drawn as required to counter suspicion. Somewhere far down the line there are volunteers chipping away at their meagre stipends to feed and transport AIDS patients under their care. The global machinery of the AIDS industry expends billions of dollars annually yet skirts the margins of society and sub-populations where the most severe effects of the epidemic are experienced and where the dynamics of the disease are best understood.

Political leadership in government is important; at the very least, it should prioritise understanding the epidemiology of the disease and use of that knowledge to actively foster multisectoral and community-level responses. Likewise, some political accountability needs to be established – at the very least, an appreciation that meddling and intransigence lead to unnecessary infection and death for hundreds of thousands of people.

The epidemic in South Africa is situated within a context of economic disadvantage and very high HIV prevalence. It may seem to be intractable and irreversible. This need not be the case. The challenge to HIV prevention in South Africa is to disrupt the sexual networks within which HIV is readily transmitted. Knowledge of the risk of having multiple and overlapping sexual partners is low; hence, this is a necessary first ingredient for a renewed political direction and multisectoral engagement.

There is equally a strong need to address the causal pathways that have exacerbated economic inequalities in the country. To date, economic empowerment of communities most affected by apartheid has been very narrowly defined. Resources have flowed to a small 'black' elite through state-sanctioned asset transfer, to individuals within the political elite and, via state employment and state-funded projects, to the creation of a 'black' middle class beholden to the government in power. Whether or not the government reconsiders its political strategy, the fracturing of South African society is becoming more apparent as the epidemic unfolds. There is a humanitarian crisis on an unprecedented scale as a result of illness and death. It will continue even if the state health system manages to expand the provision of ARVs. Treated or not, AIDS results in premature death and creates multiple burdens on all levels of society. In short, it is time to recentre political, economic and intellectual attention on how to curtail HIV/AIDS in the context of severe socio-economic inequalities and marginalisation of those most affected by the epidemic.

Notes

1. Some informal settlements have been 'formalised' through the provision of electricity to shacks, piped water to streets and sanitation services.
2. See www.pepfar.gove/press/81640.htm.
3. High viral load also occurs intermittently during the long latent phase of HIV infection as a product of co-infection with other sexually transmitted infections and also increases in the late phase of infection (see West et al. 2007).
4. Quotes from a focus group conducted by the Centre for AIDS Development, Research and Evaluation in 2008.

References

Butler, A. 2005. 'South Africa's HIV/AIDS Policy, 1994–2004: How Can It Be Explained?' *African Affairs* 104(417): 591–614.

Chigwedere, P., G. Seage, S. Gruskin, T. Lee and M. Essex. 2008. 'Estimating the Lost Benefits of Antiretroviral Drug Use in South Africa'. *Journal of Acquired Immune Deficiency Syndromes* 49(4): 410–15.

Corbett, E., B. Makamure, Y. Bun Cheungh, E. Dauya, R. Matambo and T. Bandason. 2007. 'HIV Incidence during a Cluster Randomised Trial of Two Strategies Providing Voluntary Counselling and Testing at the Workplace in Zimbabwe'. *AIDS* 21: 483–9.

Crimp, D. and A. Rolston. 1990. *AIDS Demo Graphics*. Washington: Bay Press.

Green, E., D. Halperin, V. Nantulya and J. Hogle. 2006. 'Uganda's HIV Prevention Success: The Role of Sexual Behaviour Change in the National Response'. *AIDS and Behavior* 10(4): 335–46.

Hajiyiannis, H. and W. Parker. 2008. *Talking about AIDS in an Informal Settlement: Experiences from Orange Farm, Gauteng*. Johannesburg: Centre for AIDS Development, Research and Evaluation.

Halperin, D. and H. Epstein. 2007. 'Why is HIV Prevalence So Severe in Southern Africa? The Role of Multiple Concurrent Partnerships and Lack of Male Circumcision: Implications for AIDS Prevention'. *Southern African Journal of HIV Medicine* (March): 19–27.

Hunter, M. 2002. 'The Materiality of Everyday Sex: Thinking beyond Prostitution'. *African Studies* 61(1): 99–120.

Latora, V., A. Nyamba, J. Simpore, D. Sylvette, S. Sulvere and S. Musumeci. 2006. 'Network of Sexual Contacts and Sexually Transmitted HIV Infection in Burkino Faso'. *Journal of Medical Virology* 78: 724–9.

Leclerc-Madlala, S. 2004. 'Transactional Sex and the Pursuit of Modernity'. *Social Dynamics* 29(2): 1–21.

Low-Beer, D. and R. Stoneburner. 2004. 'AIDS Communications through Social Networks: Catalyst for Behaviour Changes in Uganda'. *African Journal of AIDS Research* 3(1): 1–13.

Makhubele, M. and W. Parker. 2008. 'Growing and Sustaining Community Responses to HIV/AIDS'. A report to the Global Fund. Johannesburg: Centre for AIDS Development, Research and Evaluation.

Morris, M. and M. Kretzschmar. 2000. 'A Microsimulation Study of the Effect of Concurrent Partnerships on the Spread of HIV in Uganda'. Working paper. Population Research Institute, Pennsylvania State University.

Naidoo, P. 2003. *Youth Divided: A Review of loveLife's Y-Centre in Orange Farm.* Johannesburg: Centre for AIDS Development, Research and Evaluation.

Nattrass, N. 2004. *The Moral Economy of AIDS in South Africa.* Cambridge: Cambridge University Press.

Parker, W., B. Makhubele, P. Ntlabati and C. Connolly. 2007. *Concurrent Sexual Partnerships amongst Young Adults in South Africa: Challenges for HIV Prevention Communication.* Johannesburg: Centre for AIDS Development, Research and Evaluation.

Schneider, H. and D. Fassin. 2002. 'Denial and Defiance: A Socio-Political Analysis of AIDS in South Africa'. *AIDS* 16: S45–S51.

Schneider, H. and J. Stein. 2001. 'Implementing AIDS Policy in Post-Apartheid South Africa'. *Science and Medicine* 52: 723–73.

Shilts, R. 2000. *And the Band Played on: Politics, People and the AIDS Epidemic.* New York: St Martin's Press.

Shisana, O., T. Rehle, L. Simbayi, W. Parker, K. Zuma, A. Bhana, C. Connolly, S. Jooste and V. Pillay. 2005. *Nelson Mandela/HSRC Study of HIV/AIDS: South African National HIV Prevalence, HIV Incidence, Behaviour and Communications Survey.* Cape Town: HSRC Press.

UNAIDS (Joint United Nations Programme on HIV/AIDS). 2007. 'Global HIV Prevalence Has Levelled Off: AIDS is among the Leading Causes of Death Globally and Remains the Primary Cause of Death in Africa'. Press release. Geneva: UNAIDS.

West, G., A. Corneli, K. Best, K. Kurkjian and W. Cates. 2007. 'Focusing HIV Prevention on Those Most Likely to Transmit the Virus'. *AIDS Education and Prevention* 19(4): 275–88.

Willan, S. 2004. 'Briefing: Recent Changes in the South African Government's HIV/AIDS Policy and Its Implementation'. *African Affairs* 103: 109–17.

Conclusion

AIDS in the African State: Quo Vadis?

Segun Ige and Tim Quinlan

This book has undertaken the ambitious task of examining the coherence and disparities within and between the rhetoric(s) of African states' responses to the HIV/AIDS pandemic. The result is an analysis that focuses largely on the gap between the talk of governments about what needs to be done and what has actually happened in practice. Our purpose is not to represent a miserable and pitiful Africa – nor, we trust, is this the result of the book. The critique is sharper, we believe, for contrasting the differences that exist between those governments that have bridged or are bridging the gap and those who continue to say they are, even when the reality on the ground suggests otherwise.

The background to this critique is the continuous pressure from international agencies and local civil societies upon African governments to intervene in the HIV/AIDS crisis systemically and constructively. As the African Union's (AU's) rhetoric shows, successive African presidents, prime ministers and ministers have said that they understand the imperative, but there is some doubt (in some cases grave) based on what has happened. There are some states, Senegal and Morocco being illustrations in this book, which started well and have sustained their commitment to good effect. There are some states that started well and then lost the plot; South Africa is the primary example in this book. Uganda is cited as another example of this, in view of the government's seeming abdication of effective home-grown initiatives in the mid-2000s for a simplistic, foreign strategy and, recently, the anti-gay discourse espoused by its national legislature. There are also some states that suddenly added substantive action to the rhetoric, thereby gaining public confidence even if the measures have yet to show positive measurable outcomes – for example, Botswana, as mentioned in Chapter 1. And then there are those states that have failed miserably to date: The Gambia and South Africa, for different reasons, are the main examples in this book.

In beginning this project, we asked a number of African scholars to explore the ambivalence of African states to their citizens' welfare in the context of HIV/AIDS. As a reading of this book shows, we obtained a range of perspectives. They were predominantly pessimistic, but they were also largely cast in relation to the possibilities for effective interventions. This input led us, as editors, to find a way of framing the evidence and insights. As we describe in Chapter 1, we used Anderson's thesis that nations have potential for goodness and when they are wrong, it is temporary. That potential is evident enough in Africa, as the deliberations of the AU for the last twenty years illustrate. Likewise, the temporary nature of states being wrong is clearly evidenced in the variable record of African governments' responses to HIV/AIDS. In the case of the AU, a record of four to five years of action on the basis of nineteen years of professed commitment to the welfare of the continent's inhabitants is cause for doubt about that commitment. The source of such doubt is moral: the inhabitants of Africa, not the heads of state, have borne and continue to bear the terrible costs of the disparities within and between national responses to HIV/AIDS.

It is tempting to infer that the problem is the inordinate length of time it is taking African governments collectively to manifest their potential for goodness. However, as we discuss in Chapter 1, the historical record does not support arguments that African governments were and still are slow in responding to the pandemic. At best, the record reveals that a 'slow response' is only one aspect of the problem and even then, largely in relation to the lack of knowledge of the disease in the 1980s and the length of time for its effects to become glaringly evident. At worst, it is a misleading judgement for diverting attention away from consideration of what sort of response(s) were necessary in the past, the need for elaboration of responses as conditions and knowledge of the disease changed and, in view of the latter, the ever-changing basis for assessment and critique of government interventions.

The chapters in this book have examined these issues under the banner of the rhetoric on AIDS. The goodness and the wrongness of the responses have been explored through the lens of leadership. In Chapter 1, Ige and Quinlan summarise the tenor of the following chapters and the AU's record in terms of the limited evidence of 'transformational' leadership and the prevalence of 'incidental' leadership. In turn, these constructs led us to define the relationship between government and citizen: the former views the latter as an 'enemy'.

This assessment rests on the contributions of the other authors. Their chapters are framed by Judith Flick's consideration of three key questions for assessing leadership in Africa on the issue of HIV/AIDS in Chapter 2 and Warren Parker's encapsulation of many of the issues raised in the other chapters via an analysis that reveals the marginal-isation of civil society in the rhetoric and actions of African governments in Chapter 10.[1] Put very schematically, Fatima Harrak, John-Eudes Lengwe Kunda and Keyan Tomaselli, and Stella Nyanzi (Chapters 3, 5 and 6) explore the questions posed by Flick. Shauna Mottiar, Getnet Tadele and again, Kunda and Tomaselli (Chapters 4, 8 and 5 respectively) examine the marginalisation of civil society. The chapters of Paul Nchoji Nkwi and H. Russell Bernard and Ademola J. Ajuwon (Chapters 7 and 9) occupy the middle ground in their considerations of culture, race and ethnicity: the ever-contentious and, frequently, immediate and subliminal points of reference in public debates about the merits or demerits of governments' HIV/AIDS interventions. This schematic distinction serves only to guide the presentation below of key points that emerge from this body of work.

First, in Chapter 1 we refer to the records of Senegal and Uganda, which show that their presidents heeded the advice of scientists and used their position to mobilise their societies. In Senegal, the government enjoined Muslim clerics, recognising their social authority in a predominantly Muslim country, to join the struggle against the epidemic. In Uganda, the government supported locally conceived interventions that were effectively communicated to the populace. These were nations where appropriate answers were given to the key questions posed by Flick in Chapter 2. The national leaders appreciated the 'best' knowledge available at the time (that of science and of local culture and society), they recognised the threat to their nations, acted decisively and, as importantly, they sustained their commitment. This point is illustrated in detail in Chapter 3, in Harrak's discussion of the 'assertive leadership' that has driven Morocco's successful initiatives over time to contain the epidemic.

In contrast, the records of South Africa (Chapters 4, 5, 9 and 10) and The Gambia (Chapter 6) show what happens when such knowledge is not appreciated, indeed, is questioned by national leaders. In the case of South Africa, as we note in Chapter 1, there was a response in the early 1990s similar to that of Senegal and Uganda and, remarkably, one developed in the context of civil war. The leaders of both the apartheid regime and the liberation movement worked together in the early 1990s to create a firm foundation for the new government of 1994. However, those foundations were eroded by President Thabo Mbeki's rejection of the 'best' (ever-changing) knowledge of the times. The same effect occurred in The Gambia but via different means: through President Jammeh's abuse and manipulation of both scientists' knowledge of HIV/AIDS and local, traditional knowledge of disease and healing.

The cases of Mbeki and Jammeh reveal how not to mobilise broader society, even though they both appealed to popular opinion, local knowledge and culture. Jammeh's heavy-handed methods to gain the acquiescence of local scientific authorities and to quell dissent reveal the disingenuousness of his rhetoric. As Kunda and Tomaselli show, Mbeki's resistance/Renaissance ideology was a contradictory device for resonating with people's fears but not providing a firm basis for confronting them. In other words, Mbeki and Jammeh gave disastrous answers to the question posed by Flick in Chapter 2: 'How do leaders focus on issues that really matter to those that are entrusted to them?'

The point can be taken further. The national leaders of Senegal, Uganda and Morocco drew upon tradition and culture in very practical ways to disseminate the knowledge of scientists as well as the strategies and ideas of both local and international agencies on how to contain the HIV/AIDS epidemics in their countries. They (like Botswana's presidents in the last decade) did not seek to distract public attention as Mbeki and Jammeh did, by questioning the value of 'Western' medicine or by inferring neo-colonial conspiracies in the agendas of international agencies. Most significantly, the leaders of Senegal, Morocco (and, up to the mid-2000s, Uganda) managed not only to uphold local social and cultural norms (which would be viewed as conservative social institutions in the West), but they also introduced new information and ideas to change how local society viewed and dealt with HIV/AIDS. In sum, they epitomise a constructive joining of science and politics and, more broadly, what transformational leadership means in practice.

Second, the net effect of those governments' rhetoric was to create and open up spaces for collaboration between different agencies to determine policy and practice and subsequent interventions. This is a message that reverberates throughout this book in terms of the different chapters emphasising the necessity of civil society participation; indeed, how sustained interventions depend on the initiatives of non-governmental organisations (NGOs) and community-based organisations (CBOs) (M'boge and Doe 2004). This is the central and overt theme in Mottiar's Chapter 4. The point is made conversely in Chapters 5, 8 and 10, in terms of how marginalisation of civil society in national activities erodes the capacity of society to begin, let alone to expand upon, interventions as knowledge and conditions change. The means are diverse, but the effect is the same. Mbeki's resistance/ Renaissance ideology excluded, in effect, by playing on and endorsing people's fears. Tadele's Chapter 8, which offers a graphic discussion of societal prejudices in Ethiopia against 'gays', highlights a common widespread means. His broader dismissal of the myth that homo-sexuality is not an 'African' phenomenon is particularly pertinent in view of the homophobic discourse endorsed by the governments of Uganda and Malawi, among others. Parker (Chapter 10) reveals less obvious means in his detailed assessment of marginalisation. His critique of how the loveLife programme in South Africa is creating division between the poor and the relatively more wealthy youth in that country's slums and townships illustrates how easily interventions can negate their intent.

Third, the book highlights the power of agency; specifically, the capability of Africa's political leaders to either encourage or stultify the capacity of their nations to act constructively in the face of the epidemic. The variety of national responses, irrespective of the social and economic condition of countries, negates any suggestion that a lack of resources or poverty are substantive constraints on leaders' commitment. The point is that sound leadership depends on how leaders answer the question (modifying slightly Flick's rendition): 'How can they respect the diversity of needs and values of societies in their response to the pandemic and deal with the scale of the pandemic at the same time?'

Nkwi and Bernard's Chapter 7 and Ajuwon's Chapter 9 discuss the foundations of both constructive and negative answers described in the other chapters. For Nkwi and Bernard, constructive interventions are those that acknowledge the fact that HIV is transmitted by sexual intercourse and work with, yet also strive to modify cultural practices that exacerbate the risk of infection. Ajuwon indicates how leaders' decisions can be confounded by racist and ethnocentric interjections. In other words, debates about the scale of the pandemic in Africa and about African responses have been infused with racist explanations such that political leaders may avoid confronting facts, for fear of lending support to such explanations (for example, 'Africans are promiscuous') and/or defend cultural practices (for example, widow inheritance and virginity testing) and/or reject suggested changes, for fear of being seen to be destroying 'African culture' and heritage. Equally, the same fears can lead them to reject some behaviours as alien to Africa (for example, homosexuality).

We appreciate that this is a very schematic summary of complex cultural and behavioural dynamics within national leaders' responses to HIV/AIDS. It should be read as indicating sources for the contradictions that abound in national interventions. Nkwi, Bernard and Ajuwon show, however, that political leaders need not tie themselves in knots on these matters. Political leaders need to appreciate facts about the transmission of HIV/AIDS in Africa and, as importantly, the wealth of research and means to understand those facts. Ajuwon indicates that the field of gender studies is a vital source of pertinent information for political leaders to negotiate prejudices and for revealing how the risk of transmission is a function of relations of power, specifically, inequalities between men and women in Africa.

We have sought to show that it is possible to assess the quality of leadership within states and across Africa by comparing the diverse responses of governments. For us, it comes down to assessing whether (and, if so, how, when and why) there is a gap between government statements about what needs to be done and what has happened in practice. Again, several points can be drawn from the book's answers to these questions.

First, the diverse record of Africa's governments illustrates the difference between rhetoric and 'rhetorictery' (Booth 2004: 40), later classified as 'Rhetoric-B' (Booth 2006: 320). Rhetoric consists of 'claims that warrant belief' (323). It is a set of statements and actions that intimates substantive and logical links between knowledge of a situation, past and proposed actions and their purpose. In other words, it weaves many threads of thought and knowledge to convey clarity about a situation. 'Rhetorictery' or 'Rhetoric-B', in contrast, is the unethical performance of rhetoric, manifested in inconsistencies, in statements and actions, which beg questions about whether the threads of thought and knowledge are joined and to what end. In short, it does not convey clarity about a situation. 'Rhetorictery' is a modern term, but the phenomenon was well expressed long ago by Aristotle as 'the courage of ignorance', a phrase that aptly describes Jammeh's and Mbeki's statements and actions on HIV/AIDS.

Secondly, chapters in this book have provided many reasons for why the claims of some leaders do not warrant belief and not only on the basis of objectively discernable contradictions and inconsistencies in those claims. They have also indicated that a claim does not warrant belief if the hearers or subjects cannot see themselves in what is ostensibly a story about them. That message is graphically conveyed, for example, in Tadele's quotes from Ethiopian 'gays' about their lives in a state that views homosexuality as a crime and in Kunda and Tomaselli's argument that Mbeki's perspective on HIV/AIDS does not resonate with people's experience of it. This is the internal facet of the processes of exclusion and marginalisation, of stigma and discrimination, which are a much-publicised feature of Africans' experiences of the HIV/AIDS pandemic.

Put another way, African leaders make a mistake if they believe that appealing for an 'African' solution based on the rejection of supposedly 'non-African' agendas and values will resonate with the public in the long term. That is 'rhetorictery'. Sound rhetoric is when leaders demonstrate substantive links between the values they invoke in their pronouncements and what they do. Harrak's discussion of the national response in Morocco is testimony to this, in the monarchy's evocation of its paternal and titular responsibilities by active involvement in leading HIV/AIDS campaigns and co-ordinating government ministry policy-making bodies and, more broadly, in the co-option of Islamic clergy to broadcast the government's policies and programmes. Sound rhetoric includes also making use of modern cultural and social values, blending the old and the new. That is illustrated in the Moroccan case, in the co-option of the media and celebrities, as well as 'caravans' to reach youth on holiday at summer resorts.

It may be noted that the issues discussed above feed into broader critiques by African scholars about how African governments have exercised their mandate to create 'African' societies out of colonial legacies. We refer, for example, to Fanon (1977) and to the notion of 'Afrocentricism' (Ashante 2007). Our contribution is at the level of questioning the extent to which Africa's political leaders look towards and make use of the continent's resources. Our criticism of the AU's record, for example, is about the lack of reflection and intervention beyond reiteration of commitment. These are the grounds for asserting that this collective of heads of state generally has not demonstrated a keen understanding of what they are, what they have done and what they can do. Therefore, the AU has yet to reveal that it is an African agent capable of resolving Africans' concerns about HIV/AIDS.

Thirdly, the core reason for this book's position on the quality of leadership in Africa is that so often leaders' claims about HIV/AIDS do not warrant belief. The subliminal criticism is that the shoddy rhetoric of some leaders erodes public trust (Booth 2004: 40). It is this lack of credibility that begs questions about their commitment to public good. This inspires doubts such as their seeming ambivalence with regard to the welfare of their citizens. As we have seen, this ambivalence takes many forms in Africa. It is not a universal phenomenon across the continent. It is prevalent enough, however, to warrant global rebuke of the AU and those heads of state who have contributed to the vast death toll by AIDS in Africa.

It is this ambivalence that should continue to be the foundation for civil society in Africa – and beyond – to press for extraordinary interventions on the continent which, ironically, simply require governments 'to do what they know should be done' (St Augustine in Burke 1950: 50).

The motivation behind this book is to encourage African governments to relieve Africans of the burden they carry as a result of bad political leadership. Service delivery protests and legal suits (that have characterised civil society engagements with governments in some African states), in addition to the multitude of deaths across the continent, are an indictment of the quality of leadership in Africa. We used Anderson's idea of 'temporary wrongness' (1998: 360) to disentangle the manifold criticisms and public doubts about African governments' commitment to the welfare of their citizens that frame much of the history of HIV/AIDS in Africa. We believe we have shown that it is a useful concept for illustrating 'good' and 'bad' governments. It has helped us to show how and why some governments understood what they had to do from the start while others have found, lost and, on occasion, re-found 'the plot'. Nonetheless, thirty years into the pandemic, in post-colonial Africa, and in an era where the world knows well how to contain HIV epidemics, Africa's inhabitants may rightly ask: how long must they endure this ambivalence amongst their leaders?

Note

1. Judith Flick's questions are: How do leaders focus on issues that really matter to those that are entrusted to them; what combination of leaders and leadership is required; and how can leaders respect the diversity of needs and values of societies in their response to the pandemic and deal with the scale of the pandemic at the same time?

References

Anderson, B. 1998. *The Spectre of Nations: Nationalism, Southeast Asia and the World*. London: Verso.

Ashante, M. 2007. *An Afrocentric Manifesto: Toward an African Renaissance*. London: Polity Press.

Booth, W.C. 2004. *The Rhetoric of Rhetoric: The Quest for Effective Communication*. Oxford: Blackwell.

Burke, K. 1950. *A Rhetoric of Motives*. Berkeley: University of California Press.

Fanon, F. 1977. *The Wretched of the Earth*. New York: Grove Press.

Jost, W. (ed.). 2006. *Wayne Booth: The Essential*. Chicago: University of Chicago Press.

M'boge, F. and S. Doe. 2004. 'African Commitments to Civil Society Engagement: A Review of Eight NEPAD Countries'. AHSI Paper 6, August, African Human Security Initiative. Available at www.africanreview.org.

Contributors

Ademola J. Ajuwon earned a B.Sc. in sociology from the University of Lagos, a Master of Public Health in health promotion and education and a Ph.D. in public health education from the University of Ibadan in 2000. He is currently a professor and acting head of the Department of Health Promotion and Education at the University of Ibadan. He teaches health communication and ethics of public health research and his research interests are HIV/AIDS prevention, gender-based violence and capacity development on research ethics. He has published widely in numerous Africa-based and international journals.

H. Russell Bernard is professor emeritus of anthropology at the University of Florida. He is currently editor of the journal *Field Methods* and has served as editor for the journals *American Anthropologist* and *Human Organization*. He has also taught in Greece, Japan, Germany and England. He received his B.A. in anthropology and sociology from Queens College and his Ph.D. in anthropology from the University of Illinois. He has been a recipient of the Franz Boas Award from the American Anthropological Association as well as the University of Florida Graduate Advisor/Mentoring Award. He is a member of the United States National Academy of Sciences.

Judith Flick obtained her M.A. from the Universiteit Leiden, Hageveld. She is head of projects and planning at the Global Campaign for Education and director of projects at the Presencing Institute. She previously worked as regional global HIV and AIDS programme director and regional director at Oxfam, Great Britain, and regional director, South America. She is an experienced facilitator with extensive cross-sectoral, multilingual experience in leading cutting-edge initiatives and facilitation.

Fatima Harrak is a historian and political scientist and a graduate of the Institut d'Études Politiques in Paris and the University of London's School of Oriental and African Studies. She is a research scholar at the University Mohammed V Institute of African Studies (IAS) and served as its director from 2003 to 2008. She is the co-ordinator of a research structure at IAS dealing with religious dynamics in Africa. She has been a visiting scholar at a number of African, European and American universities and is the author of several books and numerous articles and book reviews. She has served as member and vice-chair of the scientific committee of the Council for the Development of Social Science Research on Africa (CODESRIA) and as its vice-president.

Segun Ige earned his Ph.D. from the University of Natal, Durban, specialising in rhetoric and gender. Segun has initiated a number of projects on rhetoric, one of which is the 'AIDS and the State' project that resulted in the publication of the present volume. He is editor of *African Journal of Rhetoric* and *Balagha: African Rhetoric Quarterly*. He is also founder of the African Association for Rhetoric (AAR). Aside from consulting for organisations and mentoring graduate students and academic staff, Segun is an ardent promoter of rhetoric on the African continent. His areas of interest include rhetoric, gender, presidential rhetoric and executive deliberation in multilateral organisations and leadership. He is currently consultant/CEO at JOI Consulting, a rhetoric and speech communication firm in Cape Town.

John-Eudes Lengwe Kunda holds a diploma in philosophy and anthropology, a B.A. in theology and pastoral psychology, an M.A. in communication for development and a Ph.D. in culture, communications and media studies, specialising in health and policy. He is an honorary lecturer at the University of KwaZulu-Natal and a tutor in the University of London's School of Hygiene and Tropical Medicine's distance learning programme. John has received a number of post-doctoral fellowships in HIV prevention and vaccine research. At the time of writing, he was a post-doctoral fellow at the Centre for Culture, Communications and Media Studies at the University of KwaZulu-Natal. He has worked in the field of health communication in Botswana, Namibia, Swaziland and Zambia. He has also taught communications, media studies and medical anthropology.

Shauna Mottiar is senior research fellow at the Centre for Civil Society at the University of KwaZulu-Natal. She has a Ph.D. in political studies from the University of the Witwatersrand and her research interests include civil society, social movements and social protest. She currently manages the Centre for Civil Society's philanthropy and social entrepreneurship project, focusing on the role of philanthropy in social justice and social change.

Paul Nchoji Nkwi is professor emeritus of anthropology at the University of Yaounde. He is currently also deputy vice-chancellor for academic affairs at the Catholic University of Cameroon, Bamenda. He was the founding president of the Pan African Anthropological Association (PAAA) and editor-in-chief of its journal, *The African Anthropologist*. He has been a visiting professor at Harvard, a Fulbright scholar at the University of South Carolina, visiting professor at Rhodes University and visiting scholar at the University of Leiden, The Netherlands and the University of Bergen, Norway. He received a B.A. (Honours) and a Ph.D. in anthropology from the University of Fribourg, Switzerland. He is an executive member of the International Union of Anthropological and Ethnological Sciences (IUAES).

Stella Nyanzi is a medical anthropologist who works as a research fellow at the Makerere Institute of Social Research and as a senior researcher at the Law, Gender and Sexuality Research Project at the School of Law at Makerere University. She obtained her Ph.D. from the University of London's School of Hygiene and Tropical Medicine, based on ethnographic research into the sexual and reproductive health of youths living in The Gambia. She has fifteen years of experience conducting academic research about heterosexualities in Uganda and more recently seven years focusing on The Gambia. She has published widely in journals and books. Her most recent co-authored book is *How to be a Proper Woman in the Time of AIDS*. Currently she is conducting research about the politicisation of homosexualities in Uganda by the religious right.

Warren Parker has worked globally as a consultant in the HIV/AIDS field for two decades. His focus includes development of policies and strategies, programme design, programming for social mobilisation for health and evaluation of health interventions. His Ph.D. focused on ideology and HIV/AIDS. He is an honorary lecturer in the School of Literary Studies, Media and Creative Arts at the University of KwaZulu-Natal. During the 1990s he was involved in the national 'Beyond Awareness' campaign in South Africa. He was also involved in the award-winning *Tsha Tsha* television series about young people dealing with AIDS in a small rural town. He co-founded the Centre for AIDS Development, Research and Evaluation (CADRE) in 2000 and served as executive director until early 2009.

Tim Quinlan was the research director of the Health Economics and HIV/AIDS Research Division (HEARD) from 2002 to 2010. Previously, following his training as an anthropologist at the University of Cape Town, he conducted research in the fields of environmental management and development planning at the former University of Durban-Westville. He now works independently and is a professor in a part-time post at the Athena Institute, Free University, in Amsterdam.

Getnet Tadele received his B.A., M.Sc. and Ph.D. degrees from Addis Ababa, Newcastle (Australia) and Amsterdam universities respectively. He has conducted academic and consultancy research for local and foreign universities and NGOs. In particular, he has published extensively on child abuse management, family violence and sexual abuse against children, child sex tourism, institutional childcare, alternative childcare guidelines, information management on vulnerable children, child abandonment and sexuality and HIV/AIDS. He is currently editing a forthcoming book tentatively entitled *Vulnerabilities, Impacts and Responses to HIV/AIDS in Sub-Saharan Africa*. Tadele is currently an associate professor and chair of the sociology department at Addis Ababa University, Ethiopia.

Keyan Tomaselli is director of the Centre for Communication, Media and Society at the University of KwaZulu-Natal, Durban. He helped to devise the Department of Health's two 'Beyond Awareness' campaigns and served on the minister of health's advisory committee on HIV/ AIDS and STDs between 1995 and 2000. He is co-editor, with Colin Chasi, of *Development and Public Health Communication* (2011).

Index